PHARMACOTHERAPY BEDSIDE GUIDE

NOTICE

Medicine is an ever-changing science. As new research and clinical experience broaden our knowledge, changes in treatment and drug therapy are required. The authors and the publisher of this work have checked with sources believed to be reliable in their efforts to provide information that is complete and generally in accord with the standards accepted at the time of publication. However, in view of the possibility of human error or changes in medical sciences, neither the authors nor the publisher nor any other party who has been involved in the preparation or publication of this work warrants that the information contained herein is in every respect accurate or complete, and they disclaim all responsibility for any errors or omissions or for the results obtained from use of the information contained in this work. Readers are encouraged to confirm the information contained herein with other sources. For example and in particular, readers are advised to check the product information sheet included in the package of each drug they plan to administer to be certain that the information contained in this work is accurate and that changes have not been made in the recommended dose or in the contraindications for administration. This recommendation is of particular importance in connection with new or infrequently used drugs.

PHARMACOTHERAPY BEDSIDE GUIDE

Christopher P. Martin, PharmD, MS, BCPS

Clinical Assistant Professor
College of Pharmacy, The University of Texas at Austin
Austin, Texas

Robert L. Talbert, PharmD, FCCP, BCPS, FAHA

Professor, College of Pharmacy, University of Texas at Austin
Pharmacotherapy Division
Austin, Texas
Professor, School of Medicine, University of Texas Health Science Center at San Antonio
Pharmacotherapy Education & Research Center (PERC)
San Antonio, Texas

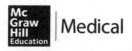

New York   Chicago   San Francisco   Lisbon   London   Madrid   Mexico City
Milan   New Delhi   San Juan   Seoul   Singapore   Sydney   Toronto

Pharmacotherapy Bedside Guide

1 2 3 4 5 6 7 8 9 0   DOC/DOC   18 17 16 15 14 13

ISBN 978-0-07-176130-7
MHID 0-07-176130-6

This book was set in Helvetica Neue by Aptara Inc.
The editors were Michael Weitz and Christina M. Thomas.
The production supervisor was Catherine Saggese.
The cover designer was Thomas DePierro.
Project management was provided Abhishan Sharma at Aptara Inc.
RR Donnelley was printer and binder.

This book is printed on acid-free paper.

Library of Congress Cataloging-in-Publication Data

Martin, Christopher P.
   Pharmacotherapy bedside guide / Christopher P. Martin, Robert L. Talbert.
      p. ; cm.
   Adapted from: Pharmacotherapy / [edited by] Joseph T. DiPiro ... [et al.]. 8th ed. c2011.
   Includes index.
   ISBN 978-0-07-176130-7 (soft cover : alk. paper) – ISBN 0-07-176130-6 (soft cover : alk. paper)
      I. Talbert, Robert L.   II. Pharmacotherapy.   III. Title.
      [DNLM: 1. Drug Therapy–Outlines.   2. Evidence-Based Medicine–Outlines.   WB 18.2]

   615.5'8–dc23

                                                              2012041055

DEDICATION

To Jennifer, Trevor and Mason, without your love and support
this would have remained an unrealized dream. —Chris

CONTENTS

CONTRIBUTORS

Andrea L. Coffee, PharmD, MBA, BCPS
Scott & White Healthcare
Temple, Texas
Section 10

Jason M. Cota, PharmD, MSc, BCPS
Assistant Professor
Department of Pharmacy Practice
University of the Incarnate
Word Feik School of Pharmacy
San Antonio, Texas
Chapters 2.1 and 2.2

Nicole L. Cupples, PharmD
Clinical Pharmacy Specialist
Psychiatry, San Antonio State Supported Living Center
San Antonio, Texas
Section 9

Phillip Lai, PharmD, BCPP
Community Care
Austin, Texas
Section 9

Cynthia Mascarenas, PharmD, MSc, BCPP
Clinical Pharmacy Specialist
South Texas Veterans Health Care System
San Antonio, Texas
Clinical Assistant Professor
Pharmacy Education and Research Center
The University of Texas Health Science Center at San Antonio
San Antonio, Texas
Section 9

Troy Moore, PharmD, MSc, BCPS
Assisant Professor
Division of Schizophrenia and Related Disorders
Department of Psychiatry
University of Texas Health Science Center at San Antonio
Clinical Pharmacy Specialist in Psychiatry
South Texas Veterans Health Care System
San Antonio, Texas
Section 9

Susan J. Rogers, PharmD, BCPS
Assistant Clinical Professor
University of Texas at Austin
Clinical Pharmacy Specialist Neurology
South Texas Healthcare System
Audie L. Murphy Veterans Hospital
San Antonio, Texas
Chapters 4.2, 4.3 and 4.4

Laurajo Ryan, PharmD, MSc, BCPS, CDE
Clinical Associate Professor
University of Texas at Austin College of Pharmacy
University of Texas Health Science Center
Pharmacotherapy Education Research Center
Department of Medicine
Austin, Texas
Chapters 3.1 and 5.2

Jeffrey S. Stroup, PharmD, BCPS, AAHIVE
Associate Professor of Medicine
Oklahoma State University Center for Health Sciences
Tulsa, Oklahoma
Section 12

John Tovar, PharmD
Associate Professor
Department of Pharmacy Practice
Feik School of Pharmacy
University of the Incarnate Word
San Antonio, Texas
Chapters 2.1 and 2.2

Nathan P. Wiederhold, PharmD
Associate Professor
University of Texas at Austin College of Pharmacy
Clinical Assistant Professor
UT Health Science Center San Antonio
San Antonio, Texas
Chapter 2.3

PREFACE

Albert Einstein is quoted as saying "If you can't explain it simply, you don't understand it well enough." Provision of good medical care is anything but simple. The decision of which pharmacotherapy to employ in the course of patient care is one of many complex decisions to be made. The clinician must simultaneously consider a multitude of variables. What are the possible benefits of the drug treatment options relative to the risk for the patient presented by this disease? What does the evidence say about which treatment should be used? How does the patient's age, gender, race, or comorbid diseases affect the choice of pharmacotherapy? What possible harm could this medicine bring to my patient? Are there any interactions with medicines this patient is already taking? Will cost of the medication be a barrier?

We developed this pharmacotherapy reference with Einstein's words in mind. The exclusive use of tables and algorithms provides a structure to display many complex variables in one place. We focused on including information that is routinely clinically relevant to produce a reference that, while not comprehensive, is high yield. Inside you will find answers to many of the questions posed above and some clinical pearls weaved in along the way. We hope this reference helps you provide the best care for your patients. Any feedback to improve future editions is most welcome.

Chris and Bob, editors

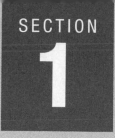

SECTION 1

Cardiology

ABBREVIATIONS

AAD	Antiarrhythmic drug	ESC	European Society of Cardiology
ACC	American College of Cardiology	GFR	Glomerular filtration rate
ACEI	Angiotensin-converting enzyme inhibitor	HCTZ	Hydrochlorothiazide
ACS	Acute coronary syndrome	HF	Heart failure
Afib	Atrial fibrillation	HR	Heart rate
AHA	American Heart Association	HTN	Hypertension
AKI	Acute kidney injury	LVEF	Left ventricular ejection fraction
ARA	Aldosterone receptor antagonist	MI	Myocardial infarction
ARB	Angiotensin receptor blocker	NCEP	National Cholesterol Education Program
BB	Beta blocker	NDCCB	Non-dihydropyridine calcium channel blocker
BP	Blood pressure		
BPM	Beats per minute	NSTEMI	Non-ST-elevation myocardial infarction
CABG	Coronary artery bypass graft	NTG	Nitroglycerin
CAD	Coronary artery disease	PCI	Percutaneous coronary intervention
CCB	Calcium channel blocker	SBP	Systolic blood pressure
CKD	Chronic kidney disease	SDC	Serum digoxin concentration
DBP	Diastolic blood pressure	SL	Sublingual
DCC	Direct current cardioversion	STEMI	ST-elevation myocardial infarction
DCCB	Dihydropyridine calcium channel blocker	UFH	Unfractionated heparin
		TdP	Torsades de Pointes
DM	Diabetes mellitus	TEE	Transesophageal echocardiogram

TABLE 1.1.1 Antihypertensive Drug Dosing

Drug (Brand)	Generic	Daily Dose Range (mg/day)	Doses Per Day
ACE Inhibitors			
Benazepril (Lotensin)	Y	10–40	1 or 2
Captopril (Capoten)	Y	12.5–150	2 or 3
Enalapril (Vasotec)	Y	5–40	1 or 2
Fosinopril (Monopril)	Y	10–40	1
Lisinopril (Prinivil, Zestril)	Y	10–40	1
Moexipril (Univasc)	Y	7.5–30	1 or 2
Perindopril (Aceon)	Y	4–16	1
Quinapril (Accupril)	Y	10–80	1 or 2
Ramipril (Altace)	Y	2.5–10	1 or 2
Trandolapril (Mavik)	Y	1–4	1
ARBs			
Candesartan (Atacand)	N	8–32	1 or 2
Eprosartan (Teveten)	N	600–800	1 or 2
Irbesartan (Avapro)	N	150–300	1
Losartan (Cozaar)	Y	50–100	1 or 2
Olmesartan (Benicar)	N	20–40	1
Telmisartan (Micardis)	N	20–80	1
Valsartan (Diovan)	N	80–320	1
BBs—β_1 Selective			
Atenolol (Tenormin)	Y	25–100	1
Betaxolol (Kerlone)	Y	5–20	1
Bisoprolol (Zebeta)	Y	2.5–10	1
Metoprolol tartrate (Lopressor)	Y	100–400	2 or 3
Metoprolol succinate (Toprol XL)	Y	50–200	1
Nebivolol (Bystolic)	N	5–20	1
BBs—Nonselective—β_1 and β_2			
Nadolol (Corgard)	Y	40–120	1
Propranolol (Inderal)	Y	160–480	2
Propranolol long-acting (Inderal LA)	Y	80–320	1
Timolol (Blocadren)	Y	10–40	1
BBs—Nonselective—β_1, β_2, and α_1			
Carvedilol (Coreg)	Y	12.5–50	2
Carvedilol phosphate (Coreg CR)	N	20–80	1
Labetalol (Normodyne, Trandate)	Y	200–800	2

(Continued)

TABLE 1.1.1 Antihypertensive Drug Dosing *(Continued)*

Drug (Brand)		Generic	Daily Dose Range (mg/day)	Doses Per Day
Calcium Channel Blockers—Dihydropyridine				
Amlodipine (Norvasc)		Y	2.5–10	1
Felodipine (Plendil)		Y	5–20	1
Isradipine (DynaCirc)		Y	5–10	2
Isradipine SR (DynaCirc SR)		Y	5–20	1
Nicardipine sustained release (Cardene SR)		Y	60–120	2
Nifedipine long acting (Procardia XL)		Y	30–90	1
Nisoldipine (Sular)		Y	10–40	1
Calcium Channel Blockers—Nondihydropyridine				
Diltiazem	(Cardizem SR, others)	Y	120–320	2
	(Cardizem CD, others)	Y	120–320	2
Verapamil	(Calan SR, Isoptin SR)	Y	120–480	1
	(Covera HS)	Y	180–480	1 at bedtime
	(Verelan PM)	Y	100–400	1 at bedtime
Central α_2 Blockers				
Clonidine (Catapress)		Y	0.1–0.8	2 or 3
Clonidine patch (Catapress—TTS)		Y	0.1–0.3	1 weekly
Methyldopa (Aldomet)		Y	250–1,000	2
Direct Arterial Vasodilators				
Minoxidil (Loniten)		Y	10–40	1 or 2
Hydralazine (Apresoline)		Y	20–100	2–4
Diuretics—Aldosterone Antagonists				
Eplerenone (Inspra)		Y	50–100	1 or 2
Spironolactone (Aldactone)		Y	25–50	1 or 2
Spironolactone/HCTZ (Aldactazide)		Y	25–50/25–50	1
Diuretics—Potassium Sparing				
Amiloride (Midamor)		Y	5–10	1 or 2
Amiloride/HCTZ (Moduretic)		Y	5–10/50–100	1
Triamterene (Dyrenium)		Y	50–100	1 or 2
Triamterene/HCTZ (Dyazide)		Y	37.5–75/25–50	1
Diuretics—Thiazides				
Chlorthalidone (Hygroton)		Y	6.25–25	1
HCTZ (HydroDiuril)		Y	12.5–25	1
Indapamide (Lozol)		Y	1.25–2.5	1

TABLE 1.1.1 Antihypertensive Drug Dosing *(Continued)*

Drug (Brand)	Generic	Daily Dose Range (mg/day)	Doses Per Day
Metolazone (Mykrox)	Y	0.5–1	1
Metolazone (Zaroxolyn)	Y	2.5–10	1
Long-Acting Nitrates[a]			
Isosorbide mononitrate (Imdur)	Y	60–240	1
Isosorbide dinitrate (Dilatrate SR)	Y	40–160	1 or 2
Peripheral Selective α_1-Blockers			
Doxazosin (Cardura)	Y	1–8	1
Prazosin (Minipress)	Y	2–20	2 or 3
Terazosin (Hytrin)	Y	1–20	1 or 2
Renin Inhibitor			
Aliskiren (Tekturna)	N	150–300	1

[a]Used primarily for angina (Table 1.2.1) or HF (Table 1.5.1), must dose to provide 12-hour nitrate-free interval.

TABLE 1.1.2 Compelling Indications and Contraindications for Antihypertensives by Class

Drug Class	Compelling Indications								Contraindications
	Angina	Afib	CAD Risk	CKD	DM	Post-MI	HF (↓ LVEF)	Stroke	
ACEIs			√	√	√	√	√	√	Angioedema, pregnancy, bilateral renal artery stenosis
ARBs				√	√		√		Pregnancy, bilateral renal artery stenosis
ARAs				√		√	√		Hyperkalemia
BBs	√	√				√	√		Severe bronchospastic disease, AV nodal block
D-CCBs	√								Severe aortic stenosis
ND-CCBs	√	√							AV nodal block, HF (↓ LVEF)
Thiazides				√		√		√	Uncontrolled gout; renal impairment is a relative contraindication

TABLE 1.1.3 Guideline Recommendations for Drug Therapy of Primary Hypertension Without Compelling Indications

Guideline	Goal and Staging	Initial Drug Treatment
Canadian Hypertension Education Program (CHEP) Canada, 2011	• Goals: <140/90 mm Hg; <130/80 mm Hg in CKD or DM • Uncomplicated: >140 SBP without compelling indications • Complicated: >140 SBP with compelling indications	• First line: thiazide, ACEI, ARB, CCB or BB • Avoid BB if age >60 • 2 drugs if SBP ≥20 mm Hg or DBP ≥10 mm Hg goal
European Society of Cardiology (ESC) Europe, 2007	• Goals: <140/90 mm Hg; <130/80 mm Hg in DM, CKD, MI, stroke, proteinuria • Grade 1: 140–159 mm Hg SBP or 90–99 mm Hg DBP • Grade 2: 160–179 mm Hg SBP or 100–109 mm Hg DBP • Grade 3: ≥ 180 mm Hg SBP or ≥ 110 mm Hg DBP	• First line: thiazide, ACEI, ARB, CCB or BB • Avoid BB (+/– thiazide) in patients with metabolic syndrome • 2 drugs if Grade 2 or 3 HTN or if high CV risk
Joint National Committee VII (JNC VII) United States, 2004	• Goals: <140/90 mm Hg; <130/80 mm Hg in CKD or DM • Stage 1: 140–159 mm Hg SBP or 90–99 mm Hg DBP • Stage 2: ≥160 mm Hg SBP or ≥100 mm Hg DBP	• First line: thiazide • Consider: ACEI, ARB, CCB or BB • 2 drugs if SBP ≥20 mm Hg or DBP ≥10 mm Hg goal • 2 drug therapy should include a thiazide
National Institute for Health and Clinical Excellent (NICE) United Kingdom, 2011	• Clinic BP Goal: <140/90 mm Hg if <80 yo; <150/90 mm Hg if ≥80 yo • Average ABPM Goal: <135/85 mm Hg if <80 yo; <145/85 mm Hg if ≥80 yo • Stage 1: ≥135 mm Hg SBP or ≥85 mm Hg DBP • Stage 2: ≥150 mm Hg SBP or ≥95 mm Hg DBP	• Step 1: ACEI or ARB if <55 yo and non-African or Caribbean origin; CCB if ≥55 yo or African or Caribbean origin • Step 2: ACEI or ARB, plus CCB • Step 3: Step 2 plus thiazide • Step 4: Step 3 plus BB, ARA, or other diuretic

• Universal recommendations:
  • Institute therapeutic lifestyle changes in every patient.
  • Tailor drug therapy based on presence of compelling indications, drug interactions, adverse reactions, and other patient-specific factors.
  • Educate patients on the importance of compliance with therapeutic lifestyle changes and drug therapy.

TABLE 1.1.4 Estimated Antihypertensive Blood Pressure Reduction by Drug Class[a]

Drug Class	Efficacy Estimate	Comments
ACEIs	−8 mm Hg SBP −5 mm Hg DBP	Represents mean SBP/DBP reduction at half maximal dose. ¼ and ½ maximum dose provides 70% and 90% maximum dose efficacy, respectively; no efficacy difference between agents (*Cochrane Database Sys Rev.* 2008, Issue 4)
ARAs	20 mmHg SBP 7 mmHg DBP	Based on spironolactone vs. placebo trials; dose response for spironolactone flat for doses ≥50 mg; efficacy estimate may be inflated (*Cochrane Database Sys Rev.* 2010, Issue 8.); eplerenone efficacy 75% of spironolactone when 100 mg doses of each compared (*Drugs.* 2003;63:1963)
α1-blockers	−8 mm Hg SBP −5 mm Hg DBP	No difference in efficacy between alpha blockers; systematic review authors feel reported efficacy an overestimate (*Cochrane Database Sys Rev.* 2009, Issue 4)
ARBs	−8 mm Hg SBP −5 mm Hg DBP	Represents mean SBP/DBP reduction at half maximal dose; ¼ and ½ maximum dose provides 70% and 80% maximum dose efficacy, respectively; no efficacy difference between agents (*Cochrane Database Sys Rev.* 2008, Issue 4)
BBs	−11 mm Hg SBP −6 mm Hg DBP	Mean SBP and DBP 2 mm Hg higher with BBs when compared directly with ACE inhibitors, ARBs, diuretics, or CCBs (*Cochrane Database Sys Rev.* 2007, Issue 1); BBs (mainly atenolol) clinical outcomes worse compared with diuretics, CCBs, ACEIs, and ARBs (*J Hypertens.* 2006;24:2131)
CCBs	−10 mm Hg SBP −5 mm Hg DBP	Based on results from dihydropyridine CCBs vs. placebo; no major differences seen between classes of CCBs (*Prog Cardio Dis.* 2004;47:34); amlodipine efficacy −12/6 mm Hg vs. placebo (Prod Info Norvasc® May 2011)
Renin inhibitor (Aliskiren)	−8 mm Hg SBP −5 mm Hg DBP	Based on aliskiren 300 mg; aliskiren 150 mg efficacy −6/3 mm Hg (*Cochrane Database Sys Rev.* 2008, Issue 4)
Thiazide diuretics	−7 mm Hg SBP	Based on a systematic review of placebo-controlled trials, mostly of HCTZ (*Am J Med.* 2009;122:290); chlorthalidone 1.5–2 times more potent than HCTZ on a mg per mg basis (*Am J Hypertens.* 2010;23:440)

[a]Efficacy estimates are derived from published meta-analyses of clinical trials comparing drugs from each class to placebo, and thus should not be used as an indication of comparative efficacy between classes.

TABLE 1.1.5 Antihypertensive Precautions and Adverse Effects by Class

Drug Class	Notable Adverse Effects (Incidence)	Comments
ACEIs	Angioedema (<1%)	More common in smokers and African-Americans
	Acute renal failure (<1%)	Elderly more sensitive; asymptomatic SCr increase common within 72 h of initiation; elevation up to 35% over baseline (if <3 mg/dL) tolerable (*Am J Kid Dis.* 2000;36:646)
	Dry cough (1–15%)	Onset as early as first day but can occur months after initiation
	Hyperkalemia (1–4%)	More common when combined with aldosterone antagonists or K^+ sparing diuretics
	Hypotension	More common in hypovolemic patients, start low dose if volume depleted
α_1-blockers	First dose phenomenon (~1%)	Characterized by orthostatic hypotension, dizziness, tachycardia; orthostasis can persist with subsequent doses; minimized by giving first dose at bedtime
	Dizziness (9–26%)	Incidence not correlated with age or BP lowering
	Weight gain (0.5%)	Thought to be from sodium and water retention; more common with high doses; may be mitigated by combining with diuretic
ARBs	Angioedema (rare)	Incidence lower than ACEIs; ARBs appear safe in patients with history of ACEI-induced angioedema (*Lancet.* 2008;372: 1174)
	Dry cough	Incidence similar to placebo in most trials; significantly lower incidence than ACEIs (*N Engl J Med.* 2008;358:1547)
	Hyperkalemia (1–4%)	Incidence similar to ACEIs (*N Engl J Med.* 2008;358:1547); more common when combined with aldosterone antagonists or K^+ sparing diuretics
	Hypotension	Appears more common than with ACEIs (*N Engl J Med.* 2008;358:1547)
ARAs	Hyperkalemia	Higher incidence has been observed with 75 mg spironolactone compared with 12.5 mg (*N Eng J Med.* 1999;341:709); median ↑ serum [K+] ~0.3 mEq/L in patients with normal renal function (*Hypertension.* 2011;57:1069; *J Am Soc Hypertens.* 2010;4:295); risk increases with declining GFR
	Gynecomastia	Incidence much higher with spironolactone than eplerenone; higher incidence with spironolactone 150 mg (52%) than 50 mg (7%) (*Am J Cardiol.* 1987;60:820)
	Menstrual abnormalities	Amenorrhea and menorrhagia have both been reported; incidence is low and poorly defined; appears dose related; higher incidence with spironolactone than eplerenone

TABLE 1.1.5 Antihypertensive Precautions and Adverse Effects by Class *(Continued)*

Drug Class	Notable Adverse Effects (Incidence)	Comments
BBs	Fatigue (2–26%)	Most common in the first week of therapy; resolves spontaneously in most patients; long-term incidence around 2% (*JAMA.* 2002;288:351)
	Sexual dysfunction	Incidence of 1 per 199 patients treated for 1 year; no difference between BBs (*JAMA.* 2002;288:351)
	Weight gain	Occurs in the first few months of therapy; median weight gain is 1.2 kg (*Hypertension.* 2001;37:250)
CCBs	Dizziness (3–10%) Headache (2–23%)	Headache and dizziness are vasodilator-related effects; both more common with dihydropyridines; headache is most common patient complaint with CCBs
	Peripheral edema (4–29%)	Incidence from lowest to highest: verapamil, diltiazem, amlodipine, nifedipine
Thiazides	Hypokalemia	Greater decline in serum [K^+] with higher doses; mean serum [K^+] decline range 0.24–0.4 mEq/L with 12.5–25 mg HCTZ and chlorthalidone (*Am J Hypertens.* 2010;23:440)
	Hyperglycemia	Glucose elevation and weight gain seen in patients with abdominal obesity taking HCTZ, more pronounced when combined with atenolol; effect not seen in patients without abdominal obesity (*Hypertension.* 2010;55:61)
	Hypercalcemia	Thiazides decrease calcium excretion and vitamin D activation but do not affect PTH (*J Endocrinol Invest.* 1989;12:531); the elevation is usually mild, lasts a few weeks and usually does not cause significant hypercalcemia on its own
	Hyperuricemia	Thiazides decrease urate excretion; does not cause gouty arthritis on its own but can exacerbate preexisting gout

TABLE 1.1.6 Selected Cardiovascular Drug Interactions[a]

Object Drug(s)	Inhibitor(s) and Inducer(s)	Comments
Contraindicated Combinations: Do not coadminister		
Sildenafil, tadalafil, vardenafil	*Isosorbide dinitrate, isosorbide mononitrate, NTG*	Combination causes profound hypotension; fatalities have been reported
Thioridazine, pimozide	*Amiodarone, conivaptan, diltiazem, dronedarone, propafenone, quinidine, ranolazine, verapamil*	Inhibit metabolism of object drugs, exacerbating QT prolongation effects and resulting in excess arrhythmia risk
Atorvastatin	Telaprevir	Telaprevir significantly increases atorvastatin concentrations, contraindicated per telaprevir (Incivek™) product labeling
Simvastatin	*Gemfibrozil*, cyclosporine	All contraindicated per product labeling. All are potent CYP 3A4 inhibitors that significantly increase simvastatin/lovastatin levels leading to risk of myopathy and rhabdomyolysis. Pravastatin is a safe alternative. Reduced risk with atorvastatin or rosuvastatin combined with gemfibrozil
Lovastatin, simvastatin	Atazanavir, boceprevir, danazol, fosamprenavir, itraconazole, lopinavir, ritonavir, posaconazole, saquinavir, telaprevir, tipranavir	
Ranolazine	Clarithromycin, ketoconazole, indinavir, itraconazole, nefazodone, nelfinavir, ritonavir, saquinavir	Contraindicated per product labeling. Potent CYP 3A4 inhibitors increase ranolazine levels and increase risk of QT prolongation and arrhythmia
Dronedarone, ranolazine	Carbamazepine, phenobarbital, phenytoin, rifampin, rifabutin, rifapentine, St. John's wort	Contraindicated per product labeling. These potent CYP 3A4 inducers decrease drug levels
Dronedarone	Cyclosporine, clarithromycin, grape fruit juice ketoconazole, itraconazole, nefazodone, ritonavir, telithromycin, voriconazole	Contraindicated per product labeling. These potent CYP 3A4 inhibitors increase dronedarone levels. Ketoconazole produces a ninefold increase in dronedarone C_{max}
Major Drug Interactions: Assess risk vs. benefit, adjust dose, or use alternative agent if possible		
Atorvastatin	Protease inhibitors, itraconazole, posaconazole	CYP 3A4 inhibitors can increase statin concentrations and increase risk of myopathy and rhabdomyolysis. Consider pravastatin or reduced dose of statin if combination unavoidable; monitor CPK levels and signs/symptoms of myopathy
Atorvastatin, lovastatin, rosuvastatin	*Gemfibrozil*, cyclosporine	
Atorvastatin, lovastatin, simvastatin	*Amiodarone*, aprepitant, clarithromycin, conivaptan, erythromycin, fluvoxamine, imatinib, ketoconazole, nefazodone, quinupristin/dalfopristin, telithromycin	

TABLE 1.1.6 Selected Cardiovascular Drug Interactions[a] *(Continued)*

Object Drug(s)	Inhibitor(s) and Inducer(s)	Comments
Fluvastatin, lovastatin, rosuvastatin, simvastatin	Fluconazole, voriconazole	Fluconazole and voriconazole are potent CYP 2C9 inhibitors. Fluconazole interaction most pronounced with high doses
Ranolazine	*Diltiazem*, erythromycin, fluconazole, grapefruit juice	Maximum dose of ranolazine is 500 mg BID in combination with these agents per product labeling.
Cyclosporine, colchicine eplerenone, ergot alkaloids sirolimus, tacrolimus, quetiapine,	*Diltiazem, verapamil*	Diltiazem and verapamil are moderate CYP 3A4 inhibitors that increase concentrations of object compounds
Digoxin	*Amiodarone*, conivaptan, itraconazole, *propafenone*, protease inhibitors, *quinidine, verapamil*	P-glycoprotein and/or CYP 3A4 inhibitors can increase serum digoxin levels
	Loop and thiazide diuretics	Hypokalemia from potassium wasting diuretics can precipitate digoxin toxicity even with normal digoxin levels. Close monitoring of serum [K+] is warranted
	Indomethacin	Decreased renal clearance of digoxin and increased serum digoxin levels have been reported when indomethacin was added to ongoing regimen with digoxin
	Clarithromycin, doxycycline, erythromycin, minocycline, tetracycline	Coadministration with these antibiotics has been reported to reduce digoxin inactivation by normal gut flora and increase digoxin levels
	St John's wort	St. John's wort induces p-glycoprotein and reduces serum digoxin levels
BBs	*Diltiazem, verapamil*	Concomitant use of BBs and NDCCBs can result in bradycardia and heart block. The interaction is more pronounced in the elderly or with left ventricular dysfunction
	Clonidine	BBs can exacerbate clonidine withdrawal from unopposed alpha stimulation
Clopidogrel	Lansoprazole, omeprazole, rabeprazole	Decreased conversion of clopidogrel to its active metabolite has been reported with these PPIs. Though controversial, some literature suggests increased risk of cardiovascular events when combined. Avoid combination if possible and consider alternative such as ranitidine

[a]Cardiovascular drugs in *italics*.

TABLE 1.1.7 Pharmacotherapy for Acute Hypertension[a]

Clinical Situation	Definitions and Goals	Treatment
Hypertensive urgency	• Definition: SBP ≥180 mm Hg or DBP ≥120 mm Hg and no symptoms of end-organ damage • Goal: Reduce to <160/100 over several hours or days (*JAMA.* 2003;289:2560)	• If on antihypertensives: Resume medications if noncompliant, increase doses of existing medications if not on max dose, add additional agent if needed • If not on antihypertensives: No evidence for superiority of any agent (*Cochrane Database Sys Rev.* 2008, Issue 1), short-acting agents such as captopril or labetalol are preferable due to rapidity of onset and ease of titration, can transition to longer acting agent once at goal, consider compelling indications and contraindications for long-term therapy (see Table 1.1.2), avoid short-acting nifedipine due to risk of reflex tachycardia
Hypertensive emergencies	• Definition: SBP ≥180 mm Hg or DBP ≥120 mm Hg and symptoms of end-organ damage • Goal and treatment vary by organ involvement	• Treatment based on specific emergency (see below) • In general, evidence in support of specific treatments is poor • Avoid nitroprusside or enalaprilat if AKI
Hypertensive encephalopathy (without stroke)	• Definition: Hypertensive emergency with papilledema or retinal hemorrhage and mental status changes, may also have AKI and proteinuria • Goal: Reduce SBP by 15–25% of the presenting value	• IV antihypertensives such as labetalol, nitroprusside, or nicardipine • Avoid nitroprusside if AKI
Ischemic stroke	• Goal: <220/120 mm Hg or <185/110 mm Hg if t-PA is to be administered (*Stroke.* 2007;38:1655)	• IV labetalol, nicardipine, or NTG
Acute pulmonary edema	• Goal: Improve symptoms of congestion and dyspnea, and improve LVEF	• IV NTG or nitroprusside along with loop diuretic • Avoid BB or hydralazine
Aortic dissection	• Goal: Reduce SBP <120 mm Hg and HR <60 bpm	• IV BB plus vasodilator such as NTG or nicardipine
Pregnancy	• Goal: Maintain SBP 140–160 mm Hg, DBP 90–105 mm Hg (*Am J Obstet Gynecol.* 2000;183:S1)	• IV labetalol or nicardipine • Nitroprusside and ACEIs contraindicated
Adrenergic crises	• Definition: Disorders associated with high sympathetic outflow, such as cocaine use, pheochromocytoma or clonidine withdrawal	• IV phentolamine drug of choice, phenoxybenzamine PO once stable and until resolution, start 10 mg BID, if needed for long term, titrate dose every few days as needed (max 100 mg/d) • Clonidine for clonidine withdrawal; if plan to d/c clonidine, taper by reducing dose by 50% every 3 days • Avoid BBs due to unopposed alpha stimulation

[a]See Tables 1.1.1 and 12.4 for dosing of PO and IV antihypertensives, respectively.

TABLE 1.2.1 Pharmacotherapy for Chronic Stable Angina and Primary Prevention of ACS

Class	Drug/Class	Indications	Dosing	Comments
Antiplatelets	Aspirin	Primary prevention	81–325 mg QD	• The potential benefit of aspirin for prevention of ischemic events must be weighed against the risk of bleeding (see 1.2.2)
	Clopidogrel (Plavix)	Primary prevention	75 mg QD	• Clopidogrel may be substituted for patients intolerant of aspirin
Antianginals	BBs	Stable angina	See Table 1.1.1	• Cardioselective BB or CCB (diltiazem, amlodipine, or felodipine) preferred, BB and CCB efficacy similar; ACC/AHA recommends BB first line due to post-MI efficacy (*J Am Coll Cardiol.* 2007;50:2264)
	Ca++ channel blockers	Stable angina	See Table 1.1.1	• Add second agent from another class (BB, CCB or LA nitrate) if continued symptoms on monotherapy
	SL NTG	Stable angina PRN	0.4 mg PRN	• BB + ACE/ARB if reduced LVEF
	Isosorbide	Stable angina	See Table 1.1.1	• CCB or isosorbide preferred for variant angina
	ACE/ARB	Stable angina with reduced LVEF	See Table 1.1.1	• Ranolazine does not effect BP; consider for patients who fail other therapies or for whom other antianginals are limited by hypotension, see Table 1.1.6 for drug interactions
	Ranolazine (Ranexa)	Stable angina	500–1,000 mg BID	
Lipid-lowering agents	Statins	Primary prevention	See Tables 1.3.1 and 1.3.5	• US National Institutes of Health NCEP approach is to treat LDL target according to risk (see Table 1.3.3)
				• UK National Health Service NICE guidelines recommend simvastatin 40 mg for any patient >40 yo at >20% 10 year risk of CAD events with no LDL target (www.nice.org.uk/CG67)
Smoking cessation	Nicotine replacement	Primary prevention	Various products (patch, gum, lozenge, spray)	• Counseling support and pharmacotherapy combined result in higher abstinence rates than either alone (*N Engl J Med.* 2002;346:506)
	Varenicline (Chantix)	Primary prevention	0.5 mg QD × 3 days, then 0.5 mg BID	• Long-acting nicotine replacement (such as the patch) can be supplemented PRN with short-acting (such as gum) for cravings
	Bupropion	Primary prevention	150 mg BID × 1 week, then 300 mg BID if tolerated	• Varenicline is associated with neuropsychiatric effects such as changes in behavior, increased aggression, depression and suicide; patients and families should be counseled to monitor for these symptoms

TABLE 1.2.2 Aspirin Efficacy and Harms in Primary Prevention

Cohort (Event Measure)	Age Group	GI Bleeding Risk (Events Per 1,000)	Estimated Events Prevented Per 1,000 Patients by 10-Year Event Risk				
			1% Risk	5% Risk	10% Risk	15% Risk	20% Risk
Males (MIs prevented per 1,000 men)	45–59 years	8	3.2	16	32	48	64
	60–69 years	24					
	70–79 years	36					
Females (strokes prevented per 1,000 women)	55–59 years	4	1.7	8.5	17	25.5	34
	60–69 years	12					
	70–79 years	18					

Source: US Preventive Services Task Force. Aspirin for the Prevention of Cardiovascular Disease: Recommendation Statement. AHRQ Publication No. 09–05129-EF-2, March 2009. Agency for Healthcare Research and Quality, Rockville, MD. http://www.uspreventiveservicestaskforce.org/uspstf09/aspirincvd/aspcvdrs.htm

FIGURE 1.2.3 Pharmacotherapy for Acute NSTEMI

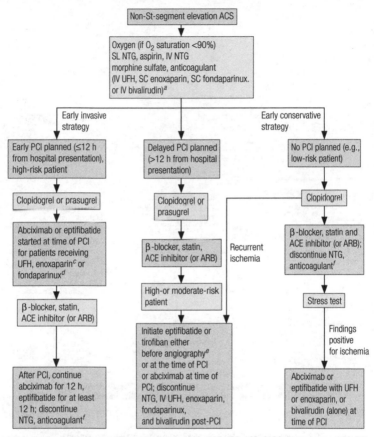

Initial pharmacotherapy for non-ST-segment elevation ACS. (ACE, ARB, ACS, CABG, IV, intravenous; NTG, PCI, SC, subcutaneous; SL, UFH).

[a]Enoxaparin, UFH, fondaparinux plus UFH, or bivalirudin for early invasive strategy; enoxaparin or fondaparinux if no angiography/PCI planned; fondaparinux or bivalirudin preferred if high risk of bleeding; UFH preferred if patients going for CABG.

[b]For patients unlikely to undergo CABG.

[c]May require an IV supplemental dose of enoxaparin.

[d]May require an IV supplemental dose of UFH.

[e]For signs and symptoms of recurrent ischemia.

[f]SC enoxaparin or UFH can be continued at a lower dose for venous thromboembolism prophylaxis.

Reprinted with permission from Spinler SA. Evolution of antithrombotic therapy used in acute coronary syndromes. In: Richardson MM, Chessman KH, Chant C, Cheng JWM, Hemstreet BA, Hume AL, et al., eds. *Pharmacotherapy Assessment Program. 7th ed.* Cardiology. Lenexa, KS: American College of Clinical Pharmacy; 2010:97–124.

FIGURE 1.2.4 Pharmacotherapy for Acute STEMI

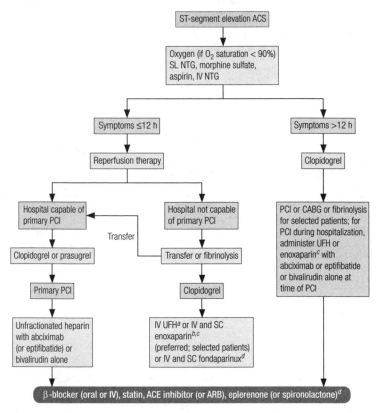

Initial pharmacotherapy for ST-segment elevation myocardial infarction. (ACS, CABG, IV, NTG, PCI, SL, UFH).
[a]For at least 48 hours.
[b]See Table 1.2.5 for dosing and specific types of patients who should not receive enoxaparin.
[c]For the duration of hospitalization, up to 8 days.
[d]For selected patients, see Table 1.2.5.
Reprinted with permission from Spinler SA. Evolution of antithrombotic therapy used in acute coronary syndromes. In: Richardson MM, Chessman KH, Chant C, Cheng JWM, Hemstreet BA, Hume AL, et al., eds. *Pharmacotherapy Assessment Program. 7th ed.* Cardiology. Lenexa, KS: American College of Clinical Pharmacy; 2010:97–124.

TABLE 1.2.5 Pharmacotherapy for Treatment and Secondary Prevention of ACS

Drug	Indications	Dosing	Comments
Antianginal Agents			
Metoprolol tartrate	ACS	5 mg IV push Q 5 min × 3	• Contraindicated for ACS in setting of cardiogenic shock
	Secondary prevention	25–150 PO mg BID	• Titrate chronic therapy to tolerated BP and HR
NTG	ACS	Initial, 5 μg/min IV, up titrate 5 μg/min every 3–5 min to response	• Avoid PVC tubing • Concomitant use of PDE-5 inhibitors may result in hypotension • Tolerance may occur with prolonged use; a nitrate-free interval is the only consistent method to avoid tolerance
Morphine	ACS	8–15 mg IV/SC every 3–4 h	• Respiratory depression may occur with large doses or rapid administration • Pruritus may occur in up to 80% of patients • Constipation may be avoided with surfactants and stimulate cathartics • Half-life of 1.5–4.5 h IV
Anticoagulants			
Bivalirudin	ACS (PCI)	0.75 mg/kg × 1, then 1.75 mg/kg/h	• Hypotension 12% • Major bleeding 3.7% • If prior UFH given, wait 30 minutes after UFH stopped to give bolus
Enoxaparin	ACS	CrCl ≥ 30 ml/min: 1 mg/kg SC Q 12 h CrCl < 30 mL/min: 1 mg.kg SC Q 24 h SC dose given 8–12 hours before PCI: 0.3 mg/kg IV	• Concomitant use in neuraxial anesthesia or LP increases risk of spinal bleeding or hematoma • Low body weight increases the risk of bleeding • Major bleeding up to 4% • Anti-Xa levels may be used in renal insufficiency to adjust doses (see 11.2.4)
	STEMI with thrombolytics	Age < 75: 30 mg IV then use ACS dosing Age ≥ 75: 0.75 mg/kg Q 12 h	
Fondaparinux	ACS	<50 kg: 5 mg SC for 5–9 days 50–100 kg: 7.5 mg SC for 5–9 days	• Concomitant use in neuraxial anesthesia or LP increases risk of spinal bleeding or hematoma • Body weight less than 50 kg increased risk of bleeding • Cr_{CL} 50–80 mL/min ↓ clearance 25% • Cr_{CL} 30–50 mL/min ↓ clearance 40% • Cr_{CL} <30 mL/min contraindicated

(Continued)

TABLE 1.2.5 Pharmacotherapy for Treatment and Secondary Prevention of ACS (Continued)

Drug	Indications	Dosing	Comments
UFH	ACS	60–70 units/kg IV bolus (maximum 5,000 units) then 12–15 units/kg/h	• Concurrent use of other antithrombotics increases the risk of bleeding • Thrombocytopenia 1–10% • Monitor anti-Xa levels 0.3–0.7 units/mL or aPTT 1.5–2 times normal • PCI target ACT: 250–350 s (200–250 with GPIIb/IIIa) • Discontinue if platelet counts drop below 100,000 cells/mcL or is reduced by 50%; consider measuring antibodies and give bivalirudin
Intravenous Antiplatelet Agents			
Abciximab	ACS w/ PCI	0.25 mg/kg IV bolus (over 5 min) followed by 0.125 mg/dk/min (max 10 µg/min) IV infusion for 12 h	• Do not remove arterial sheath unless aPTT <50 sec or ACT <175 sec • Thrombocytopenia 2.5–5.2%
Eptifibatide	ACS w/ PCI	IV bolus 180 µg/kg actual body weight (max 22.6 mg) followed by 2 µg/kg ABW/min (max 15 mg/h) until discharge, CABG or PCI	• Cr$_{CL}$ <50 mL/min reduce maintenance dose to 1 µg/kg/min • Target aPTT 50–70 sec or ACT 200–300 sec • Major bleeding 1.3–10.8% • See other warnings for abciximab
Tirofiban	ACS w/ PCI	0.4 µg/kg/min IV for 30 min then 0.1 µg/kg/min for 12–24 h after angioplasty or atherectomy	• Tirofiban inferior to abciximab for 30 day mortality, recurrent MI or revascularization (N Engl J Med. 2001;344) • Maintain catheter sheath for femoral access until 3–4 h after D/C heparin and ACT <180 sec and aPTT <45 sec
Oral Antiplatelet Agents			
Aspirin	ACS	325 mg load, then 81–325 mg/day	• May worsen asthma in patients with hypersensitivity • Bleeding more common in elderly, alcohol use and other gastric irritants and antithrombotic agents
	Secondary prevention	81–325 mg QD	
Clopidogrel	ACS	300–600 mg load, then 75 mg QD	• Reduced function CYP 2C19 alleles may reduce activation to active metabolite; genetic testing is available • Premature discontinuation may increase the risk of CV events especially in PCI with DES • TTP has been rarely reported, typically occurs around 2 weeks after initiation • Discontinue 5–7 days prior to major surgical procedures • Major bleeding 0.8–3.7%
	Secondary prevention	75 mg QD	

TABLE 1.2.5 Pharmacotherapy for Treatment and Secondary Prevention of ACS *(Continued)*

Drug	Indications	Dosing	Comments
Prasugrel	ACS	60 mg load, then 10 mg QD (5 mg QD if < 60 kg)	• Increased bleeding in BW <60 kg and concurrent use of other antithrombotics
	Secondary prevention	10 mg/day	• Not recommended for age >75 years, prior stroke • Major bleeding 2.2% • Discontinue 7 days prior to major procedures
Ticagrelor	ACS	180 mg load, then 90 mg BID	• Aspirin dose should be <100 mg/day, otherwise effectiveness is reduced
	Secondary prevention	90 mg BID	• Discontinue 5 days prior to major procedures • Potent inhibitors/induces of CYP3A may increase bleeding risk or reduce effectiveness • Dyspnea 13.8% • Ventricular pauses 6% • Major bleeding 4.5% • Concomitant doses of lovastatin or simvastatin >40 mg should be avoided
Thrombolytics[a]			
Alteplase	ACS-STEMI	>67 kg: total dose 100 mg IV, give 15 mg IV bolus, 50 mg over 30 min, then 35 mg over 60 min <67 kg: 15 mg IV bolus, then 0.75 mg/dk over 30 min, the 0.5 mg/kg over 60 min	• Do not exceed 100 mg • Use of a protocol posed in ED/CICU allows for rapid determination of exclusion criteria and less confusion in dosing • Minimize arterial and venous punctures
Reteplase	ACS-STEMI	10 units IV bolus, 2 doses given 30 min apart	• Minimize arterial and venous puncture • Overall bleeding 15–21% • Intracranial hemorrhage 0.8%
Tenecteplase	ACS-STEMI	<60 kg: give 30 mg 60–69 kg: give 35 mg 70–79 kg: give 40 mg 80–89 kg: give 45 mg >90 kg: give 50 mg	• Minimize arterial and venous punctures • Major bleeding 4.7% • Administer as single IV bolus over 5 sec

[a]Contraindications for all thrombolytics: Bleeding diathesis, cerebrovascular accident (stroke), severe uncontrolled HTN (SBP >180 mm Hg), active internal bleeding, intracranial or intraspinal surgery within 2 months, intracranial neoplasm, AV malformation or aneurysm.

TABLE 1.3.1 Approximate LDL Lowering by Statins According to the Rule of 7[a]

Approximate LDL Decline	Statin Dose (% LDL Reduction)						
	Fluvastatin	Pravastatin	Lovastatin	Pitavastatin	Simvastatin	Atorvastatin	Rosuvastatin
20%	20 mg (22%)	10 mg (22%)	10 mg (21%)				
27%	40 mg (25%)	20 mg (26–32%)	20 mg (24–27%)	1 mg (31–32%)	10 mg (30%)		
34%		40 mg (30–34%)	40 mg (30–31%)	2 mg (36–39%)	20 mg (38%)	10 mg (35–39%)	
41%			80 mg (40–42%)	4 mg (41–45%)	40 mg (29–41%)	20 mg (43%)	
48%					80 mg (36–47%)	40 mg (50%)	10 mg (46–52%)
55%						80 mg (55–60%)	20 mg (47–55%)
62%							40 mg (55–63%)

Sources: (1) Roberts WC. The rule of 5 and the rule of 7 in lipid lowering by statin drugs. *Am J Cardiol.* 1997;80(1):106–107. (2) Statin dose comparison. Pharmacist's Letter/Prescriber's Letter 2009 (Full update October 2011);25(8):250801.

[a]Rule of 7—When the dose of a statin is doubled, the expected additional LDL decline is around 7% regardless of statin or dose. The expected HDL increase is around 7%.[1]

TABLE 1.3.2 Comparative Antidyslipidemic Efficacy by Drug Class

Drug Class	LDL	HDL	TG
HMG-CoA reductase inhibitors (statins)	↓ to ↓↓↓	↑	↓↓
Fibrates	↑	↑↑	↓↓
Niacin	↓↓	↑↑↑	↓↓
Omega-3 fatty acids (fish oil)	↓	↑↑	↓↓
Bile acid sequestrants	↓	↑	↓ to ↑
Ezetimibe	↓	↑	↓
Vytorin (ezetimibe + atorvastatin)	↓↓	↑	↓
Advicor (ER niacin + simvastatin)	↓↓ to ↓↓↓	↑↑	↓↓

Approximate changes in each lipid component:
↑ –5–10%
↑↑ 10–30%
↑↑↑ 30–60%

TABLE 1.3.3 NIH NCEP Adult Treatment Panel III LDL Cholesterol Goals

Risk Category	LDL Goal (mg/dL)	LDL Level at Which to Initiate TLC (mg/dL)	LDL Level at Which to Consider Drug Therapy (mg/dL)
High risk: CHD or CHD risk equivalents	<100 mg/dL (optional goal: <70)	≥100	≥100
(10-year risk >20%)			(<100 mg/dL; consider drug options)[a]
Moderately high risk: 2+ risk factors	<130	≥130	≥130
(10-year risk >10–20%)			(100–129: consider drug options)
Moderate risk: 2+ risk factors (10-year risk <10%)	<130	≥130	≥160
Lower risk: 0–1 Risk factor[b]	<160	≥160	≥190
			(160–189: LDL-lowering drug optional)

LDL indicates low-density lipoprotein; CHD, coronary heart disease.

Reproduced with permission from Talbert RL. Dyslipidemia. In: Talbert RL, DiPiro JT, Matzke GR, Posey LM, Wells BG, Yee GC, eds. *Pharmacotherapy: A Pathophysiologic Approach.* 8th ed. New York, NY: McGraw-Hill; 2011:chap 28. http://www.accesspharmacy.com/content.aspx?aID=7974214. Accessed June 5, 2012, Table 28–8, page 372.

[a]Some authorities recommend use of LDL-lowering drugs in this category if an LDL cholesterol level of <100 mg/dL cannot be achieved by TLC. Others prefer use of drugs that primarily modify triglycerides and HDL (e.g., nicotinic acid or fibrates). Clinical judgment also may call for deferring drug therapy in this subcategory.

[b]Almost all people with 0–1 risk factor have a 10-year risk <10%; thus, 10-year risk assessment in people with 0–1 risk factor is not necessary.

TABLE 1.3.4 Antidyslipidemic Drug Dosing

Drug	Products	Dosing
HMG-CoA Reductase Inhibitors (Statins)[a]		
Atorvastatin (Lipitor)	10, 20, 40, and 80 mg tablets	10–80 mg QD
Fluvastatin (Lescol)	20, 40 mg capsules, 80 mg tablets	20–80 mg QD
Lovastatin (Mevacor)	20, 40 mg tablets	20–40 mg QD
Pitavastatin (Livalo)	1, 2, 4 mg tablets	1–4 mg QD
Pravastatin (Pravachol)	10, 20, 40 mg tablets	10–40 mg QD
Simvastatin (Zocor)	5, 10, 20, 40, and 80 mg tablets	5–40 mg QD, 80 mg in selected patients[b]
Rosuvastatin (Crestor)	5, 10, 20, 40 mg tablets	5–40 mg QD
Fibrates		
Gemfibrozil (Lopid)	600 mg tablet	600 mg BID
Fenofibrate	54 and 160 mg tablets (Lofibra, generic); 40, 120 mg tablets (Fenoglide); 50, 160 mg tablets (Triglide); 48, 145 and 160 mg tablets (Tricor)	40–160 mg QD
Bile Acid Sequestrants		
Cholestyramine (Questran)	4 g packets	4–8 g BID-TID
Colestipol (Colestid)	5 g packets	5–30 g QD (or in divided doses)
Colesevelam (Welchol)	3.75 g packet; 625 mg tablets	1875–3750 g QD
Other		
Ezetimibe (Zetia)	10 mg tablets	10 mg QD
Niacin IR	50, 100, 250, and 500 mg tablets (various brands)	2–3 g TID
Niacin ER (Niaspan)	500, 750, and 1000 mg tablets	500–2000 mg QHS
Omega-3 fatty acids (Lovaza, Omacor)	1 g capsules containing EPA 465 mg/DHA 375 mg	4 g QD (or divided BID)
Combination Products		
Niacin ER + lovastatin (Advicor)	Niacin/lovastatin 500/20, 750/20 and 1,000/20 mg tablets	500/20–1,000/20 mg QHS
Simvastatin + ezetimibe (Vytorin)	Simvastatin/ezetimibe 10/10, 20/10, 40/10, and 80/10 mg	10/10–80/10 mg QD

Reproduced with permission from Talbert RL. Dyslipidemia. In: DiPiro JT, Talbert RL, Matzke GR, Posey LM, Wells BG, Yee GC, eds. *Pharmacotherapy: A Pathophysiologic Approach.* 8th ed. New York, NY: McGraw-Hill; 2011:chap 28. Table 28–12.

[a]Choose dose according to desired LDL decline, see Table 1.3.1 for LDL lowering by statin dose.

[b]Due to high risk of myopathy, 80 mg should be reserved only for patients who have a history of tolerating this dose.

TABLE 1.3.5 Adverse Effects of Antidyslipidemic Drugs

Drug Class	Common AEs	Serious AEs
HMG-CoA reductase inhibitors (statins)	• Myalgia (20–30%), myositis (3–5%) • GI upset (up to 14%) • URI symptoms (8.3%) • UTI (up to 8%)	• Hepatotoxicity (0.2–2.3%) • Myopathy, rhabdomyolysis (~3.5 cases/1 million prescriptions); rarely leading to acute renal failure (*Ann Intern Med.* 2009;150:858) • Tendon rupture (in women, OR 3.76; not reported in men, *J Cardiovas Pharmacol.* 2009;53:401)
Fibrates	• Abdominal pain (4.6–9.8%) • Acute appendicitis (1.2%) • Indigestion (19.6%)	• Hepatotoxicity (3–4% LFT elevation) • Myopathy (2.3/10,000 person-years), rhabdomyolysis • Cholelithiasis (1–4%) • Potential reduction in renal function
Niacin	• Flushing >80%, itching, rash • Abdominal pain (4–9%) • Dry skin	• Hepatotoxicity • Peptic ulcer (uncommon) • Arrhythmias (rare)
Omega-3 fatty acids (fish oil)	• Abdominal bloating (3%) • Belching/burping (4%) • Urticarial rash	• Bleeding, thrombocytopenia (uncommon) • Hypersensitivity (uncommon)
Bile acid sequestrants	• Constipation, abdominal pain, flatulence, nausea (up to 30%) • Steatorrhea (uncommon)	• Fecal impaction, intestinal obstruction (uncommon) • Fat-soluble vitamin deficiency (uncommon–large doses, long duration, mostly children) • Osteoporosis (rare, long-term use)
Ezetimibe	• Diarrhea (2.5–4%), arthralgia (2.6–3%), URI symptoms • Myalgia (3.8%)	• Anaphylaxis, angioedema (rare) • Pancreatitis, hepatitis (0.5–3% elevated LFTs), cholelithiasis (uncommon)

FIGURE 1.4.1 Management Algorithm for Atrial Fibrillation

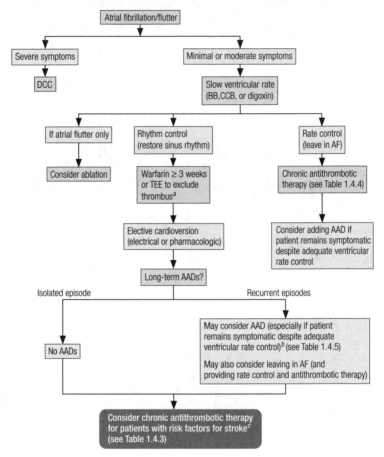

[a]If AF <48 hours, anticoagulation prior to cardioversion is unnecessary; may consider TEE if patient has risk factors for stroke.

[b]Ablation may be considered for patients who fail or do not tolerate 1 AAD.

[c]Chronic antithrombotic therapy should be considered in all patients with AF and risk factors for stroke regardless of whether or not they remain in sinus rhythm.

Reproduced with permission from Sanoski CA, Bauman JL. The arrhythmias. In: DiPiro JT, Talbert RL, Matzke GR, Posey LM, Wells BG, Yee GC, eds. *Pharmacotherapy: A Pathophysiologic Approach. 8th ed.* New York, NY: McGraw-Hill; 2011:chap 25, Figure 25–5, page 284

TABLE 1.4.2 Rate and Rhythm Control Agents for Atrial Fibrillation

Drug	Comments
Rate Control	
BBs	• BBs or NDCCBs preferred for most patients with persistent or permanent afib, diltiazem supressed heart rate better than carvedilol, metoprolol, or verapamil in a small prospective trial (*Am J Cardiol.* 2013;111:225.)
NDCCBs (diltiazem or verapamil)	• Avoid NDCCBs in HF with reduced LVEF; avoid IV NDCCBs or BBs in patients with hypotension or acute HF (*Circulation.* 2006;114:e257.)
Digoxin	• Digoxin effect on rate control delayed average 9.5 h after initiation (*Am J Cardiol.* 1993;72:567.); digoxin induce rate control abrogated by sympathetic stimulation during exercise (*Drugs.* 2003;63:1489) • Consider adding digoxin to BB or NDCCB if rate not controlled with a single agent (*Circulation.* 2006;114:e257.)
Rhythm Control	
Amiodarone	• Amiodarone superior to flecainide, propafenone, and sotalol in preventing afib recurrence (*N Engl J Med.* 2000;342:913)
Dronedarone	• Amiodarone preferred if concurrent HF; sotalol or dronedarone preferred if concurrent ischemic heart disease (*Europace.* 2010;12:1360)
Dofetilide	
Flecainide	• Avoid flecainide and propafenone if concurrent ischemic heart disease due to proarrhythmia risk (*N Engl J Med.* 1991;324:781); avoid dronedarone in advanced HF due to higher death rates (*N Engl J Med.* 2008;358:2678.)
Propafenone	
Sotalol	• Amiodarone is slightly more effective than dronedarone but dronedarone may have fewer side effects (*J Cardiovasc Electrophysiol.* 2010;21:597; *J Am Coll Cardiol.* 2009;54:1089)

TABLE 1.4.3 Antithrombotic Agents for Atrial Fibrillation

Drug	Dosing	Comments
Antiplatelet Agents		
Aspirin (various strengths)	81–325 mg OD	• Clopidogrel may be considered for aspirin intolerant patients for whom antiplatelet therapy is indicated (see Table 1.4.4 for antiplatelet indications)
Clopidogrel (Plavix) 75 mg tablet	75 mg QD	• Aspirin plus clopidogrel may be considered for patients with afib who cannot take anticoagulation for reasons other than bleeding risk (*Chest.* 2012;141:e601S) but should be otherwise avoided due to a lack of efficacy and higher bleeding risk (*Lancet.* 2004;364:331, *N Engl J Med.* 2012;367:817.)

(Continued)

TABLE 1.4.3 Antithrombotic Agents for Atrial Fibrillation *(Continued)*

Drug	Dosing	Comments
Anticoagulants		
Warfarin	Dose to target INR: • 2–3 nonvalvular afib • 2–3 aortic bileaflet mechanical valve • 2.5–3.5 all other mechanical valves	• Dabigatran was better than warfarin for prevention of stroke (RR 0.73, 95% CI 0.52–0.81) with similar bleeding outcomes in patients with intermediate stroke risk (mean $CHADS_2$ = 2.1) (*N Engl J Med*. 2010;363:1875)
Dabigatran (Pradaxa) 150 mg tablets	150 mg BID if CrCl >30 mL/min 75 mg BID if CrCl 15–30 mL/min	• Rivaroxaban was noninferior to warfarin for both efficacy and bleeding end points in patients with high stroke risk (mean $CHADS_2$ = 3.5) (*N Engl J Med*. 2011;365:883)
Rivaroxaban (Xarelto) 15 and 20 mg tablets	20 mg QD if CrCl >50 mL/min 15 mg QD if CrCl 15–50 mL/min Give with evening meal	• Apixiban was similar to warfarin for prevention of ischemic stroke (HR 0.92 95% CI 0.74–1.13) with lower hemorrhagic stroke (0.24% vs 0.47%, p<0.001, *N Engl J Med*. 2011;365:92)
Apixiban (Eliquis) 2.5 amd 5 mg tablets	5 mg BID 2.5 mg BID if age ≥80, weight ≤60 kg or SCr ≥1.5 mg/dL	

TABLE 1.4.4 Guideline Recommendations for Antithrombotic Therapy for Primary Stroke Prevention in Atrial Fibrillation[a]

Recommended Therapy	ACC/AHA Guidelines 2006	ESC Guidelines 2012
No therapy	• Age <60 + no heart disease	• Absence of risk factors
Antiplatelet therapy	• Age <60 + heart disease but no other risk factors • Age 60–74 + no heart disease and no other risk factors	• No recommendations
Either antiplatelet therapy or oral anticoagulation	• Male + age >75 + no heart disease and no other risk factors	• 1 clinically relevant nonmajor risk factor
Oral anticoagulation	• Age 60–74 + CAD or DM • Male + age >75 + any other risk factors • Any other patient with moderate or high risk factors	• $CHADS_2$ ≥2
Risk factor definitions	Weaker risk factors: • Female gender, age 60–74, CAD, thyrotoxicosis Moderate-risk factors: • Age ≥75, HTN, HF, DM High-risk factors: • Previous stroke, TIA or embolism (anywhere), mitral stenosis, prosthetic heart valve	Clinically relevant nonmajor risk factors: • HF or LVEF ≤40%, HTN, DM, female gender, age 65–74, vascular disease Major risk factors: • Previous stroke, TIA, or systemic embolism, age ≥75 $CHADS_2$ score: • 1 point each for presence of Age >75, HTN, DM, or HF • 2 points for previous stroke or TIA • Add points together to get score

[a]See Table 4.1.3 for secondary prevention recommendations.

TABLE 1.4.5 Antiarrhythmic Drug Indications and Dosing

Drug	Class	Indications	Dosing
Intravenous Agents			
Adenosine		SVT termination	6 mg IV bolus × 1, repeat 12 mg IV bolus × 2 if rhythm fails to terminate
Amiodarone	III	AF termination	5 mg/kg IV over 30 min, followed by infusion of 1 mg/min for 6 h, then 0.5 mg/min
		Stable VT	150 mg IV over 10 min, followed by infusion of 1 mg/min for 6 h, then 0.5 mg/min
		Pulseless VT/VF	300 mg IV/IO push (can give additional 150 mg IV/IO push if persistent VT/VF), followed by infusion of 1 mg/min for 6 h, then 0.5 mg/min
Diltiazem	IV	PSVT; AF (rate control)	0.25 mg/kg IV over 2 min (may repeat with 0.35 mg/kg IV over 2 min), followed by infusion of 5–15 mg/h
Digoxin		AF (rate control)	0.25 mg IV Q 2 h up to 1.5 mg total load, then 0.125–0.25 mg IV QD (if NPO)
Esmolol	II	AF (rate control)	0.5 mg/kg (500 µg/kg) IV over 1 min load, then 0.50 mg/kg/min (50 µg/kg/min) infusion
Ibutilide	III	AF (termination)	1 mg IV over 10 min (may repeat if needed)
Lidocaine	Ib	Stable VT	1–1.5 mg/kg IV push (can give additional 0.5–0.75 mg/kg IV push every 5–10 min if persistent VT (maximum cumulative dose = 3 mg/kg), followed by infusion of 1–4 mg/min (1–2 mg/min if liver disease or HF)
		Pulseless VT/VF	1–1.5 mg/kg IV/IO push (can give additional 0.5–0.75 mg/kg IV/IO push every 5–10 min if persistent VT/VF (maximum cumulative dose = 3 mg/kg), followed by infusion of 1–4 mg/min (1–2 mg/min if liver disease or HF)
Metoprolol	II	AF (rate control)	5 mg IV Q 5 min load, then 1.25–5 mg IV Q 6 h
Procainamide	Ia	AF (termination); stable VT	15–18 mg/kg IV over 60 min, followed by infusion of 1–4 mg/min
Sotalol	III	AF (patients unable to take PO sotalol)	75–150 mg IV once or twice daily (infused over 5 h)
Verapamil	IV	PSVT; AF (rate control)	2.5–5 mg IV over 2 min (may repeat up to maximum cumulative dose of 20 mg); can follow with infusion of 2.5–10 mg/h

(Continued)

TABLE 1.4.5 Antiarrhythmic Drug Indications and Dosing *(Continued)*

Drug	Class	Indications	Dosing
Oral agents			
Amiodarone	III	VT prevention	400 mg PO BID-TID up to 10 g total load, then 200–400 mg PO QD
		AF (rhythm control)	400 mg PO BID-TID up to 10 g total load, then 100–200 PO mg QD
Digoxin		AF (rate control)	0.25 mg PO Q 2 h up to 1.5 mg total load, then 0.125–0.5 mg PO QD
Diltiazem	IV	AF (rate control), SVT	IR formulation 30–60 mg PO Q 6 h or SR formulation 60–120 mg PO BID or CD formulation 120–240 mg PO QD
Disopyramide	Ia	AF (rhythm control), SVT prevention	100–150 mg PO Q 6 h or SR formulation 200–300 mg PO Q 12 h
Dofetilide	III	AF (rhythm control)	0.5 mg (500 μg) PO Q 12 h
Dronedarone	III	AF (rhythm control)	400 mg PO Q 12 h
Flecainide	Ic	AF (rhythm control), SVT/VT prevention	50–200 mg PO Q 12 h
Metoprolol	II	AF (rate control)	25–100 mg PO BID
Mexiletine	Ib	VT prevention	150–300 mg PO Q 8–12 h
Propafenone	Ic	AF (rhythm control), SVT/VT prevention	IR formulation 150–300 mg PO Q 8 h or SR formulation 225–425 mg PO Q 12 h
Quinidine	Ia	SVT/VT prevention	Quinidine sulfate 200–300 mg PO Q 6 h or quinidine gluconate 324–648 mg PO Q 8–12 h
Sotalol	III	AF (rhythm control), VT prevention	80–160 mg PO Q 12 h
Verapamil	IV	AF (rate control)	120–480 mg PO QD

TABLE 1.4.6 Antiarrhythmic Drug Adverse Effects

Drug	Adverse Effects
Disopyramide	Anticholinergic symptoms (dry mouth, urinary retention, constipation, blurred vision), nausea, anorexia, TdP, HF, conduction disturbances, ventricular arrhythmias
Procainamide	Hypotension, TdP, worsening HF, conduction disturbances, ventricular arrhythmias
Quinidine	Cinchonism, diarrhea, abdominal cramps, nausea, vomiting, hypotension, TdP, worsening HF, conduction disturbances, ventricular arrhythmias, fever, hepatitis, thrombocytopenia, hemolytic anemia
Lidocaine	Dizziness, sedation, slurred speech, blurred vision, paresthesia, muscle twitching, confusion, nausea, vomiting, seizures, psychosis, sinus arrest, conduction disturbances
Mexiletine	Dizziness, sedation, anxiety, confusion, paresthesia, tremor, ataxia, blurred vision, nausea, vomiting, anorexia, conduction disturbances, ventricular arrhythmias

TABLE 1.4.6 Antiarrhythmic Drug Adverse Effects *(Continued)*

Drug	Adverse Effects
Flecainide	Blurred vision, dizziness, dyspnea, headache, tremor, nausea, worsening HF, conduction disturbances, ventricular arrhythmias
Propafenone	Dizziness, fatigue, bronchospasm, headache, taste disturbances, nausea, vomiting, bradycardia or AV block, worsening HF, ventricular arrhythmias
Amiodarone	Tremor, ataxia, paresthesia, insomnia, corneal micro-deposits, optic neuropathy/neuritis, nausea, vomiting, anorexia, constipation, TdP (<1%), bradycardia or AV block (IV and oral use), pulmonary fibrosis, liver function test abnormalities, hepatitis, hypothyroidism, hyperthyroidism, photosensitivity, blue-gray skin discoloration, hypotension (IV use), phlebitis (IV use)
Dofetilide	Headache, dizziness, TdP
Dronedarone	Nausea, vomiting, diarrhea, serum creatinine elevations, bradycardia, TdP (<1%)
Ibutilide	Headache, TdP, hypotension
Sotalol	Dizziness, weakness, fatigue, nausea, vomiting, diarrhea, bradycardia or AV block, TdP, bronchospasm, worsening HF

Reproduced with permission from Sanoski CA, Bauman JL. The arrhythmias. In: DiPiro JT, Talbert RL, Matzke GR, Posey LM, Wells BG, Yee GC, eds. *Pharmacotherapy: A Pathophysiologic Approach.* 8th ed. New York: McGraw-Hill; 2011:chap 25, Table 25–3, page 280.

TABLE 1.5.1 Pharmacotherapy for Heart Failure with Reduced LVEF

Drug (Brand)	Starting Dose	Target Dose	Comments
ACE Inhibitors			
Captopril (Capoten)	6.25–12.5 mg TID	50 mg TID	• ACEIs listed have proven survival benefit in clinical trials at target doses and are recommended for most patients (*J Card Fail.* 2010;16:475; *J Am Coll Cardiol.* 2009; 53:e1)
Enalapril (Vasotec)	2.5–5 mg BID	10–20 mg BID	
Lisinopril (Zestril, Prinivil)	2.5–5 mg QID	20–40 mg QD	• If cannot achieve target dose, there is evidence of equal benefit with lower doses of lisinopril (*Circulation.* 1999;100:2312) and enalapril (*Eur Heart J.* 1998;19:481)
Ramipril (Altace)	1.25–2.5 mg BID	5 mg BID	• Double dose every 1–2 weeks to target dose or as tolerated
			• Use lower starting dose in renal insufficiency or volume depletion
			• Monitor SCr, serum [K⁺], and BP w/in 1–2 weeks of start or dose change
			• Effect on SCr variable: SCr ↓ in 24%, SCr ↑ <30% in 41%, SCr ↑ >30% in 35% of pts. w/ enalapril (*Am J Cardiol.* 1992;70:479)

(Continued)

**TABLE 1.5.1 Pharmacotherapy for Heart Failure with Reduced
LVEF** *(Continued)*

Drug (Brand)	Starting Dose	Target Dose	Comments
ARBs			
Candesartan (Atacand)	4 mg QD	32 mg QD	• Recommended if intolerant of ACEI (*J Card Fail.* 2010;16:475); appear safe in patients with ACEI-induced angioedema (*Lancet.* 2008;372:1174–1183)
Losartan (Cozaar)	12.5 mg QD	100 mg QD	
Valsartan (Diovan)	40 mg BID	160 mg BID	• Better outcomes but more side effects if added to ACEI and BB (*Lancet.* 2003;362:767), consider adding ARB to target dose ACEI + beta if poorly controlled but not if recent MI (*J Card Fail.* 2010;16:475)
			• Same monitoring and titration as ACEIs (see above)
BBs			
Bisoprolol (Zebeta)	1.25 mg QD	10 mg QD	• BBs listed have proven survival benefit in clinical trials at target doses and are recommended for most patients (*J Card Fail.* 2010;16:475; *J Am Coll Cardiol.* 2009;53:e1)
Carvedilol (Coreg)	3.125 mg BID	25 mg BID	
Carvedilol-controlled release (Coreg CR)	10 mg QD	80 mg QD	• Do not initiate BBs in decompensated patients
Metoprolol succinate (Toprol XL)	12.5–25 mg QD	200 mg QD	• Double dose every 2 weeks until to target dose or as tolerated
			• Reduce dose if HR ≤55 bpm
			• Fatigue common when first initiated, resolves after 1 week in most patients
			• Metoprolol tartrate (Lopressor) should not be substituted for metoprolol succinate due to poor outcomes (*Lancet.* 2003;362:7)
Aldosterone Antagonists			
Eplerenone (Inspra)	25 mg QD	50 mg QD	• Consider in symptomatic patients despite target dose ACEI + BB (*J Card Fail.* 2010;16:475; *J Am Coll Cardiol.* 2009;53:e1)
Spironolactone (Aldactone)	12.5–25 mg	50 mg QD	• Not recommended if serum [K$^+$] >5 mEq/L or CrCl <30 mL/min (*J Am Coll Cardiol.* 2009;53:e1) due to risk of hyperkalemia
			• Median ↑ serum [K$^+$] ~0.3 mEq/L in patients with normal renal function (*Hypertension.* 2011; 57:1069; *J Am Soc Hypertens.* 2010; 4:295)
			• Gynecomastia, amenorrhea, or menorrhagia are rare side effects, incidence is dose related, and much more common with spironolactone.

TABLE 1.5.1 Pharmacotherapy for Heart Failure with Reduced LVEF *(Continued)*

Drug (Brand)	Starting Dose	Target Dose	Comments
Vasodilators			
Hydralazine (Apresoline)	25 mg QID	75 mg TID	• Hydralazine + isosorbide combination can be considered in patients poorly controlled on ACEI or ARB + BB or ACEI/ARB intolerant patients (*J Am Coll Cardiol.* 2009;53:e1)
Isosorbide dinitrate (Isordil)	20 mg TID	40 mg TID	• Patients of African-American decent already on ACEI or ARB + BB in particular may benefit from combination (*N Engl J Med.* 2004;35:2049) • Increase to target dose over 2 weeks if tolerated • Provide 10–12 h nitrate-free interval with isosorbide to prevent tolerance
Positive Inotrope			
Digoxin (Lanoxin)	Dose is based on IBW, CrCl, and SDC monitoring (see Table 1.5.2); typical dose is 0.125 mg QD		• Consider for symptomatic patients despite optimal ACEI + BB or for patients with afib in need of rate control (*J Card Fail.* 2010;16:475) • Improves quality of life and prevents hospitalization but not mortality (*N Engl J Med.* 1997;336:525) • Discontinuation of digoxin associated with clinical deterioration (*N Engl J Med.* 1993;329:1) • Target SDC 0.5–0.9 ng/mL; SDC >1.0 ng/mL is associated with poor outcomes (*J Card Fail.* 2010;16:475); SDC should be measured 1 week after initiation or dose change and at least 6 h after receiving a dose
Loop Diuretics			
Furosemide (Lasix)	Based on symptoms, typical dose 20–40 mg QD		• May be required chronically to manage congestion and edema
Torsemide (Demadex)	Based on symptoms, typical dose 10–20 mg QD		• Dose conversion: furosemide 20 mg ≈ torsemide 10 mg ≈ bumetanide 0.5 mg
Bumetanide (Bumex)	Based on symptoms, typical dose 0.5–1 mg QD		• Furosemide 20 mg PO ≈ 10 mg IV (2:1 ratio); torsemide PO ≈ IV • The bioavailability of furosemide is highly variable between individuals; torsemide may offer more consistent absorption and efficacy in some patients (*J Am Coll Cardiol.* 2009;53:e1) • Though these drugs are structurally related to sulfonamide antibiotics, the risk of allergic cross-sensitivity appears low or negligible in patients with sulfonamide allergy (*Ann Pharmacother.* 2005;39:290)

TABLE 1.5.2 Digoxin Dosing for Heart Failure

IBW (kg)	CrCl (mL/min)	Dose (mg)
50	20	0.125 every other day
	40	0.125 every other day
	60	0.125 daily
	80	0.125 daily
	100	0.125 daily
	120	0.25 daily[a]
55	20	0.125 every other day
	40	0.125 every other day
	60	0.125 daily
	80	0.125 daily
	100	0.125 daily
	120	0.25 daily[a]
60	20	0.125 every other day
	40	0.125 every other day
	60	0.125 daily
	80	0.125 daily
	100	0.125 daily
	120	0.25 daily[a]
65	20	0.125 every other day
	40	0.125 daily
	60	0.125 daily
	80	0.125 daily
	100	0.25 daily[a]
	120	0.25 daily[a]
70	20	0.125 every other day
	40	0.125 daily
	60	0.125 daily
	80	0.125 daily
	100	0.25 daily[a]
	120	0.25 daily
75	20	0.125 daily
	40	0.125 daily
	60	0.125 daily
	80	0.125 daily
	100	0.25 daily[a]
	120	0.25 daily
80	20	0.125 daily
	40	0.125 daily
	60	0.125 daily
	80	0.25 daily[a]
	100	0.25 daily[a]
	120	0.25 daily

TABLE 1.5.2 Digoxin Dosing for Heart Failure *(Continued)*

IBW (kg)	CrCl (mL/min)	Dose (mg)
85	20	0.125 daily
	40	0.125 daily
	60	0.125 daily
	80	0.25 daily[a]
	100	0.25 daily
	120	0.25 daily
90	20	0.125 daily
	40	0.125 daily
	60	0.25 daily[a]
	80	0.25 daily[a]
	100	0.25 daily
	120	0.25 daily

Dosing in this table targets a SDC of 0.7 ng/mL; check level 1 week after initiation or dose change. See reference below for full dosing nomogram.
Source: Baumann JL, DiDomineco RJ, Marlos V, Fitch M. A method of determining the dose of digoxin for heart failure in the modern era. *Arch Int Med.* 2006;166:2539–2545.
[a]May consider alternating 0.125 mg and 0.25 mg every other day.

TABLE 1.5.3 Pharmacotherapy for Special Situations in Heart Failure Patients

Clinical Situation	Pharmacotherapy
Systolic dysfunction and ischemic heart disease	• Treat risk factors: hyperlipidemia, HTN, and smoking cessation • ACEI + BB at target doses • Nitrates for symptomatic angina despite BB therapy • Amlodipine or felodipine for symptomatic angina despite nitrate and BB
Asymptomatic systolic dysfunction and HTN	• ACEI + BB at target doses • If BP remains >130/80 mm Hg, add thiazide diuretic • Add amlodipine or felodipine, if still elevated
Symptomatic systolic dysfunction and HTN	• ACEI + BB at target doses • If BP >130/80 mm Hg, add aldosterone antagonist or ISDN + hydralazine, titrate to target doses • If BP remains >130/80 mm Hg despite target dose ACEI + BB + aldosterone antagonist + ISDN + hydralazine, add amlodipine or felodipine
HF with preserved LVEF	• ACEI or ARB if concurrent DM • BB if history of MI, HTN, or rate control for afib • NDCCB if afib and intolerant of BB • ACEI or ARB if none of the above apply • Loop diuretics for volume overload

Source: Lindenfeld J, Albert NM, Boehmer JP, et al. Executive summary: HFSA 2010 comprehensive heart failure practice guideline. *J Card Fail.* 2010;16:475–539.

FIGURE 1.5.4 Diuretic Algorithm for Treatment of Volume Overload in Acute Decompensated Heart Failure

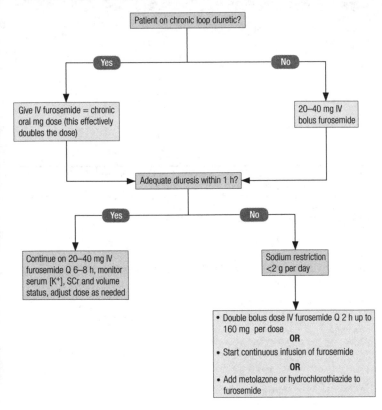

TABLE 1.5.5 Pharmacotherapy for Acute Decompensated Heart Failure

Drug (Brand)	Dosing		Comments
Diuretics			
Furosemide (Lasix)	Bolus dose	Initial: 20–40 mg IV	• See also Figure 1.5.4 for algorithm
		Max: 160–200 mg IV	• High doses required in renal impairment from reduced renal tubular concentrations
	Continuous infusion	Initial: 40 mg load, then 5 mg/h	• Symptom improvement is through venodilation and ↓ PCWP in addition to diuretic effect
		Max: 40 mg/h	
Torsemide (Demadex)	Bolus dose	Initial: 10–20 mg IV	• Acute worsening can occur from overreduction of preload or from systemic vasoconstriction due to neurohormonal activation
		Max: 200 mg IV	
	Continuous infusion	Initial: 20 mg load, then 5 mg/h	• Monitor serum [K^+], SCr, and fluid status
		Max: 20 mg/h	
Vasodilators			
NTG	Initial: 5 µg/min Titration: ↑ 5–10 µg/min Q 5 min until response Typical dose: 35–200 µg/min		• Preferred vasodilator in most patients • ↓ LV filling pressure through venodilation • Up to 20% of patients develop resistance to NTG (*J Am Coll Cardiol.* 2009;53:e1); this can occur within a few hours of initiation
Nitroprusside	Initial: 0.1–0.2 µg/kg/min Titration: ↑ 0.1–0.2 µg/kg Q 5–10 min until response Typical dose: 0.5–3 µg/kg/min		• Avoid in patients with renal impairment due to potential cyanide toxicity • ↓ preload, ↓ afterload, and ↑ CO through both arterial and venous dilation • Useful in patients with both volume overload and HTN
Nesiritide	2 µg/kg load, then 0.01 µg/kg/min infusion		• Use is limited by expense, risk of hypotension, and lack of mortality benefit (*N Engl J Med.* 2011;365:32) • May be helpful in patients without hypotension or cardiogenic shock who do not respond to NTG or nitroprusside.
Inotropes			
Dobutamine	Initial: 0.25–0.5 µg/kg/min, titrate to response Maximum: 20 µg/kg/min		• Inotropes can be considered in patients with ↓ LVEF ↓ peripheral perfusion (low output syndrome) who also have ↓ SBP and/or are refractory to vasodilators (*J Card Fail.* 2010;16:475)
Milrinone	Infusion: 0.1–0.5 µg/kg/min initial, titrate to response up to 0.75 µg/kg/min Renal impairment: Start dose at low end of range		• Continuous BP and ECG monitoring is recommended (*J Card Fail.* 2010;16:475) • Tachycardia and ↑ myocardial O_2 demand are concerns with dobutamine; prolonged hypotension and thrombocytopenia with milrinone; risk of arrhythmia with both

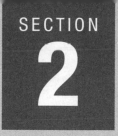

ABBREVIATIONS

ABLC	Amphotericin B lipid complex	IE	Infective endocarditis
ABM	Acute bacterial meningitis	LAMB	Liposomal amphotericin B
AUC	Area under the curve	MIC	Minimum inhibitory concentration
CAP	Community-acquired pneumonia	MRSA	Methicillin-resistant *Staphylococcus aureus*
CDI	*Clostridium difficile* infection		
CLSI	Clinical Laboratory Standards Institute	MSSA	Methicillin-susceptible *Staphylococcus aureus*
CNS	Central nervous system	PCN	Penicillin
CRBSI	Catheter-related bloodstream infections	PD	Pharmacodynamic
		PK	Pharmacokinetic
CSF	Cerebrospinal fluid	SSTI	Skin and soft tissue infections
EUCAST	European Committee on Antimicrobial Susceptibility Testing	TBW	Total body weight
		UTIs	Urinary tract infections
HAP	Hospital-acquired pneumonia	VRE	Vancomycin-resistant enterococcus
IAI	Intra-abdominal infections		
IBW	Ideal body weight	WBC	White blood cell

TABLE 2.1.1 General Approach to Infectious Diseases

Step One: Confirm Infection

General signs and symptoms of infection include:
- Temperature >101°F (>100.4°F in some instances)
- WBC >10 with bands >10%
- Assess for infection-specific signs/symptoms according to algorithms

Step Two: Perform Diagnostic Tests/Workup

- Ensure that cultures are obtained from the site of the infection *BEFORE* antimicrobial administration
- Gram stain and morphology from culture results may further guide empiric selection
- Assess for severity of infection according to algorithms

Step Three: Start Empiric Therapy

- Review list of likely infectious etiologies according to the algorithms that are largely based on infection site
- Start empiric therapy according to algorithms (base decision on local susceptibility patterns where possible, that is, antibiograms)
- Empiric antimicrobial dosing recommendations can be found in Tables 2.1.2 – 2.1.4

Step Four: Reevaluate/Monitor Response to Therapy

- Check for resolution of signs and symptoms
- Follow-up culture results/susceptibilities and note MIC when available
- Use Table 2.1.5 to monitor for adverse effects associated with selected empiric therapy and serum concentrations where necessary

Step Five: Streamline/Narrow Antimicrobial Therapy

- Use the most narrow spectrum antimicrobial that is susceptible from culture results
- If MIC results are available, consider selecting an antimicrobial with an MIC well below susceptibility breakpoints found in Table 2.1.6 (NOTE: MICs should *NOT* be compared across different antimicrobials)

Example

Blood Culture Results: *Escherichia coli*

	S/I/R	MIC	Breakpoint		
Ampicillin/sulbactam	R	>32	≤8	←	Resistant
Cefepime	S	2	≤8	←	Compare MIC = 2 to breakpoint ≤8 ("very susceptible")
Ceftriaxone	I	2	≤1	←	Intermediate
Ciprofloxacin	S	1	≤1	←	Compare MIC = 1 to breakpoint ≤1 ("susceptible")

In the example above, cefepime may be selected over ciprofloxacin because the cefepime MIC is well below the cefepime *E. coli* susceptibility breakpoint of ≤8. The ciprofloxacin MIC is equivalent to the ciprofloxacin *E. coli* susceptibility breakpoint of ≤1. If ciprofloxacin is more appropriate for the patient, then PK–PD dosing should be optimized (Table 2.1.3).

TABLE 2.1.2 Dosing Regimens for Commonly Selected Intravenous Antimicrobials

Class/Drugs	Infection/Pathogen	Normal Dose (Infusion Time)	Recommended Dosing for Susceptible Organisms		
			CrCl 30–59	CrCl 15–29	CrCl <15 or IHD
PCNs					
Ampicillin	All indications/organisms	2 g Q 4 h (0.5-h infusion)	2 g Q 6 h	2 g Q 8 h	2 g Q 12 h
		4 g Q 8 h (8-h infusion)[a]	—	—	—
Ampicillin/sulbactam	All indications/organisms	3 g Q 6 h (0.5-h infusion)	No Δ	3 g Q 12 h	3 g Q 24 h
Nafcillin	CRBSI/MSSA	2 g Q 4 h (0.5-h infusion)	No Δ	No Δ	No Δ
		12 g (24-h continuous infusion)[a]			
Oxacillin	CRBSI/MSSA	2 g Q 4 h (0.5-h infusion)	No Δ	No Δ	No Δ
		12 g (24-h continuous infusion)[a]			
PCN G[a]	ABM/susceptible organisms	24 mU (24-h continuous infusion)	No Δ	12 mU	8 mU
	IE/CRBSI/Enterococcus	20 mU (24-h continuous infusion)	No Δ	10 mU	5 mU
	IE/viridans (MIC ≤0.125)	18 mU (24-h continuous infusion)	No Δ	10 mU	5 mU
	IE/viridans (MIC 0.25–0.5)	24 mU (24-h continuous infusion)	No Δ	12 mU	8 mU
Piperacillin/tazobactam	All indications/Pseudomonas	4.5 g Q 6 h (0.5-h infusion)	Normal dosing if CrCl >40, if CrCl 30–40 dose for CrCl 15–29	3.375 g Q 6 h	2.25 g Q 6 h
	All indications/Escherichia coli	3.375 g Q 6 h (0.5-h infusion)		2.25 g Q 6 h	2.25 g Q 8 h
Cephalosporins					
Cefazolin	CRBSI/IE/osteo/MSSA	2 g Q 8 h (IV push)	2 g Q 12 h	1 g Q 12 h	1 g Q 24 h
	IAV/E. coli	2 g Q 8 h (IV push)	2 g Q 12 h	1 g Q 12 h	1 g Q 24 h
	SST/MSSA	1 g Q 8 h (IV push)	1 g Q 12 h	1 g Q 24 h	500 mg Q 24 h
	UTI/E. coli	1 g Q 8 h (IV push)	1 g Q 12 h	1 g Q 24 h	500 mg Q 24 h

Cefepime	All indications/*Pseudomonas*	2 g Q 8 h (0.5-h infusion)	2 g Q 12 h	2 g Q24 h	1 g Q24 h
	IAI/*E. coli*	2 g Q 12 h (0.5-h infusion)	2 g Q 24 h	1 g Q 24 h	500 mg Q 24 h
	UTI/all organisms	1 g Q 12 h (0.5-h infusion)	1 g Q 24 h	500 mg Q 24 h	250 mg Q 24 h
Cefotaxime	CAP/*Streptococcus pneumoniae*	2 g Q 8 h (IV push)	No Δ	2 g Q 12 h	2 g Q24 h
	CNS/*S. pneumoniae*	2 g Q 4 h (IV push)	2 g Q 6 h	2 g Q 8 h	2 g Q24 h
	IAI/*E. coli*	2 g Q 8 h (IV push)	No Δ	2 g Q 12 h	2 g Q24 h
	UTI/*E. coli*	1 g Q 8 h (IV push)	No Δ	1 g Q 12 h	1 g Q24 h
Cefotetan	Pelvic inflammatory disease[b]	2 g Q 12 h (0.5-h infusion)	No Δ	2 g Q 24 h	2 g Q 48 h
Cefoxitin	IAI/all organisms	2 g Q 6 h (0.5-h infusion)	2 g Q 8 h	2 g Q 12 h	2 g Q 24 h
Ceftaroline	All indications/organisms	600 mg Q 12 h (1-h infusion)	400 mg Q 12 h	300 mg Q 12 h	200 mg Q 12 h
Ceftriaxone	CAP/*S. pneumoniae*	1 g Q 24 h (IV push)	No Δ	No Δ	No Δ
	CNS/*S. pneumoniae*	2 g Q 12 h (IV push)			
	All indications/*E. coli*	1 g Q 24 h (IV push)			
	IE/viridans streptococci	2 g Q 24 h (IV push)			
	Osteo/all organisms	2 g Q 24 h (IV push)			
Carbapenems					
Doripenem	All indications/organisms	500 mg Q 8 h (1-h infusion)	250 mg Q 8 h	250 mg Q 12 h	250 mg Q 24 h
Ertapenem	All indications/organisms	1 g Q 24 h (0.5-h infusion)	No Δ	No Δ	500 mg Q 24 h
Imipenem/ cilastatin	All indications/organisms	500 mg Q 6 h (0.5-h infusion)	500 mg Q 8 h	250 mg Q 6 h	250 mg Q 12 h
		1 g Q 8 h (0.5-h infusion)	500 mg Q 6 h	500 mg Q 8 h	500 mg Q 12 h
Meropenem	ABM/All organisms	2 g Q 8 h (0.5-h infusion)	2 g Q 12 h	1 g Q 12 h	1 g Q 24 h
	Non-CNS indications	1 g Q 8 h (0.5-h infusion)	1 g Q 12 h	500 mg Q 12 h	500 mg Q 24 h

(Continued)

TABLE 2.1.2 Dosing Regimens for Commonly Selected Intravenous Antimicrobials *(Continued)*

Class/Drugs	Infection/Pathogen	Normal Dose (Infusion Time)	Recommended Dosing for Susceptible Organisms			
			CrCl 30–59	CrCl 15–29	CrCl <15 or IHD
Fluoroquinolones						
Ciprofloxacin	HAP/*Pseudomonas*	400 mg Q 8 h (1-h infusion)	No Δ	400 mg Q 12 h	400 mg Q 24 h
	IAI/All organisms	400 mg Q 12 h (1-h infusion)	No Δ	400 mg Q 24 h	200 mg Q 24 h
	UTI/All organisms	200 mg Q 12 h (1-h infusion)	No Δ	200 mg Q 24 h	200 mg Q 24 h
Levofloxacin	CAP/HAP/IAI/All organisms	750 mg Q 24 h (1-h infusion)	750 mg Q 48 h	500 mg Q 48 h	500 mg Q 48 h
	UTI/all organisms	250 mg Q 24 h (1-h infusion)	No Δ	No Δ	250 mg Q 48 h
Moxifloxacin	All indications/organisms	400 mg Q 24 h (1-h infusion)	No Δ	No Δ	No Δ
Macrolides						
Azithromycin	All indications/organisms	500 mg Q 24 h (1-h infusion)	No Δ	No Δ	No Δ
Tetracyclines						
Doxycycline	All indications/organisms	100 mg Q 12 h (1-h infusion)	No Δ	No Δ	No Δ
Minocycline	All indications/organisms	100 mg Q 12 h (1-h infusion)	No Δ	No Δ	No Δ
Aminoglycosides[c]						
Amikacin[d]	HAP/*Pseudomonas*	15–20 mg/kg (IBW) Q 24 h (1-h infusion)	15 mg/kg (IBW) Q 36 h	10 mg/kg (IBW) Q 48 h	Not recommended
	UTI/*Pseudomonas*	10 mg/kg (IBW) Q 24 h (1-h infusion)	10 mg/kg (IBW) Q 36 h	7 mg/kg (IBW) Q 48 h	Not recommended
Gentamicin[e]	HAP/*Pseudomonas*	7 mg/kg (IBW) Q 24 h (1-h infusion)	5 mg/kg (IBW) Q 36 h	5 mg/kg (IBW) Q 48 h	Not recommended
	UTI/*Pseudomonas*	3 mg/kg (IBW) Q 24 h (1-h infusion)	3 mg/kg (IBW) Q 36 h	3 mg/kg (IBW) Q 48 h	Not recommended
Tobramycin[e]	HAP/*Pseudomonas*	7 mg/kg (IBW) Q 24 h (1-h infusion)	5 mg/kg (IBW) Q 36 h	5 mg/kg (IBW) Q 48 h	Not recommended
	UTI/*Pseudomonas*	3 mg/kg (IBW) Q 24 h (1-h infusion)	3 mg/kg (IBW) Q 36 h	3 mg/kg (IBW) Q 48 h	Not recommended

Other					
Aztreonam[f]	ABM/IAI/HAP/gram negative	2 g Q 6 h	No Δ	1 g Q 6 h	500 mg Q 6 h
	UTI/gram negatives	1 g Q 12 h	No Δ	500 mg Q 12 h	250 mg Q 12 h
Colistin[g,h]	All indications/organisms	2.5 mg/kg (IBW) Q 12 h (0.5-h infusion)	2 mg/kg (IBW) Q 12 h	1.25 mg/kg (IBW) Q 12 h	1.25 mg/kg (IBW) Q 24 h
Clindamycin	All indications/organisms	600 mg Q 6–8 h	No Δ	No Δ	No Δ
Daptomycin	SSTI/MRSA	4 mg/kg (TBW) Q 24 h (1-h infusion)	No Δ	4 mg/kg (TBW) Q 48 h	6 mg/kg (TBW) after IHD session
	IE/MRSA	6 mg/kg (TBW) Q 24 h (1-h infusion)	No Δ	6 mg/kg (TBW) Q 48 h	6 mg/kg (IBW) Q 24 h
Linezolid	All indications/organisms	600 mg Q 12 h (1-h infusion)	No Δ	No Δ	No Δ
Metronidazole	All indications/organisms	500 mg Q 8 h (0.5-h infusion)	No Δ	No Δ	No Δ
Tigecycline	All indications/organisms	100 mg × 1, 50 mg Q 12 h (1-h infusion)	No Δ	No Δ	No Δ
Vancomycin[i]	Serious infections/organisms	15–20 mg/kg (TBW) Q 8–12 h	15–20 mg/kg (TBW) Q 12 h	15 mg/kg (TBW) Q 24 h	15 mg/kg (TBW) Q 48 h
	SSTIs/All organisms	1 g Q 12 h	1 g Q 12 h	1 g Q 24 h	1 g Q 48 h

[a] Suggested for outpatient parenteral antimicrobial therapy or ease of inpatient administration.

[b] Should be used in combination with doxycycline; not recommended for intra-abdominal infections due to ↑ Bacteroides fragilis resistance.

[c] Dose should be individualized based on therapeutic drug monitoring; consider pharmacy pharmacokinetic consult.

[d] Draw peak level 1 h after end of infusion of first dose (goal peak = 40–50) and 8–10 h random level (goal 8–10 h random <10).

[e] Draw peak level 1 h after end of infusion of first dose (goal peak = 20–25) and 8–10 h random level (goal 8–10 h random <5).

[f] Generally reserved for gram-negative infections (including Pseudomonas) in PCN-allergic patients; cross-sensitivity may occur with ceftazidime allergy.

[g] Considerable debate on doses >300 mg/day; in CrCl >70, may consider 480 mg × 1; 24 h later start 240 mg Q 8 h (Antimicrob Agents Chemother. 2009;53:3430).

[h] May consider 5–8 mg/kg (IBW) × 1; 24 h later start maintenance dose in mg of 2 × (1.5 × CrCl + 30) Q 12 h (Antimicrob Agents Chemother. 2011;55:3284).

[i] Expert recommendation for 8 mg/kg for MIC >1 or VRE.

[j] Draw trough prior to 4th dose (goal trough 15–20 mg/L) (Alternative goal trough 10–15 mg/L for SSTIs).

TABLE 2.1.3 Alternative Pharmacokinetic–Pharmacodynamic Dosing Strategies for Commonly Selected Intravenous Antimicrobials[a]

Class/Drugs	MIC (mg/L)					
	≤0.5	1	2	4	8	16
PCNs[b]						
Piperacillin/tazobactam	2.25 g Q 8 h (4 h)	2.25 g Q 8 h (4 h)	2.25 g Q 8 h (4 h)	3.375 g Q 8 h (4 h)	3.375 g Q 8 h (4 h)	3.375 g Q 8 h (4 h)
	4.5 g Q 8 h (0.5 h)	4.5 g Q 8 h (0.5 h)	4.5 g Q 8 h (0.5 h)		13.5 g (24 h)	13.5 g (24 h)
Cephalosporins[c]						
Cefazolin	1 g Q 8 (0.5 h)	1 g q8 (0.5 h)	2 g Q 8 h (0.5 h)	—	—	
	3 g (24 h)	4 g (24 h)	6 g (24 h)			
Cefepime	1 g Q 12 h (0.5 h)	1 g Q 8 h (0.5 h)	1 g Q 8 h (3 h)	2 g Q 8 h (3 h)	2 g Q 8 h (3 h)	—
		2 g Q 12 h (0.5 h)	2 g Q 8 h (0.5 h)			
Carbapenems[d]						
Meropenem	500 mg Q 8 h (1 h)	500 mg Q 8 h (3 h)	500 mg Q 8 h (3 h)	1 g Q 8 h (3 h)	—	—
		500 mg Q 6 h (1 h)	1 g Q 8 h (1 h)			

Aminoglycosides[a]						
Amikacin	10 mg/kg Q 24 h (1 h)	10 mg/kg Q 24 h (1 h)	10 mg/kg Q 24 h (1 h)	15 mg/kg Q 24 h (1 h)	20 mg/kg Q 24 h (1 h)	—
Gentamicin	5 mg/kg Q 24 h (1 h)	5 mg/kg Q 24 h (1 h)	7 mg/kg Q 24 h (1 h)	—	—	—
Tobramycin	5 mg/kg Q 24 h (1 h)	5 mg/kg Q 24 h (1 h)	7 mg/kg Q 24 h (1 h)	—	—	—
Other						
Vancomycin[f]	15–20 mg/kg Q 8-12 h (goal trough 10–15) 30–40 mg/kg 24-h continous infusion (goal level 10–15)	15–20 mg/kg Q 8-12 h (goal trough 15–20) 30–40 mg/kg 24-h continous infusion (goal level 15–20)	30–40 mg/kg 24-h continous infusion (goal level 25–30)	—	—	—

[a]Assuming normal kidney and liver function; infusion times are in parentheses.

[b]PK–PD goal is to keep concentrations above the MIC >50% of the time; general strategies include ↓ dose more frequently, extended or continuous infusion time.

[c]PK–PD goal is to keep concentrations above the MIC >60% of the time; general strategies include ↓ dose more frequently, extended or continuous infusion time.

[d]PK–PD goal is to keep concentrations above the MIC >40% of the time; general strategies include ↓ dose more frequently, extended or continuous infusion time.

[e]PK–PD goal is to achieve C_{max}: MIC 8–10; general strategy includes once-daily dosing for high C_{max} and trough <1 mg/L to decrease nephrotoxicity.

[f]PK–PD goal is to achieve AUC: MIC >400; general strategy includes ↑ total daily dose if trough levels <10 mg/L.

TABLE 2.1.4 Dosing Regimens for Commonly Selected Oral Antimicrobials

Class/Drugs	Infection/Pathogen	Normal	CrCl 30–59	CrCl 15–29	CrCl <15 or IHD
			Recommended Dosing for Susceptible Organisms		
PCNs					
Amoxicillin	CAP/*Streptococcus pneumoniae*	1 g Q 8 h	No Δ	500 mg Q 8 h	500 mg Q 24 h
Amoxicillin–clavulanate	CAP/*S. pneumoniae*	875 mg Q 12 h	No Δ	500 mg Q 12 h	500 mg Q 24 h
PCN VK	Pharyngitis/*S. pyogenes*	500 mg Q 6 h	500 mg Q 8 h	500 mg Q 12 h	500 mg Q 12 h
Cephalosporins					
Cefdinir	CAP/*S. pneumoniae*	300 mg Q 12 h	No Δ	300 mg Q 24 h	300 mg Q 48 h
Cefpodoxime	All indications/organisms	200 mg Q 12 h	No Δ	200 mg Q 24 h	200 mg Q 48 h
Cefprozil	All indications/organisms	500 mg Q 12 h	No Δ	500 mg Q 24 h	500 mg Q 24 h
Ceftibuten	All indications/organisms	400 mg Q 24 h	200 mg Q 24 h	100 mg Q 24 h	400 mg Q 48 h
Cefuroxime	All indications/organisms	400 mg Q 12 h	No Δ	No Δ	400 mg Q 24 h
Cephalexin	SSTI/*S. pyogenes*	500 mg Q 6–12 h	500 mg Q 8 h	500 mg Q 12 h	500 mg Q 24 h
Fluoroquinolones					
Ciprofloxacin	UTI/*Escherichia coli*	250 mg Q 12 h	No Δ	No Δ	250 mg Q 24 h
Levofloxacin	CAP/*S. pneumoniae*	750 mg Q 24 h	750 mg Q 48 h	500 mg Q 48 h	500 mg Q 48 h
	UTI/*E. coli*	250 mg Q 24 h	No Δ	No Δ	250 mg Q 48 h
Moxifloxacin	All indications/organisms	400 mg Q 24 h	No Δ	No Δ	No Δ
Tetracyclines					
Doxycycline	All indications/organisms	100 mg Q 12 h	No Δ	No Δ	No Δ
Minocycline	All indications/organisms	100 mg Q 12 h	No Δ	No Δ	No Δ

Macrolides					
Azithromycin	All indications/organisms	500 mg Q 24 h	No Δ	No Δ	No Δ
Clarithromycin	All indications/organisms	500 mg Q 12 h	No Δ	250 mg Q 12 h	250 mg Q 24 h
Telithromycin	CAP/all organisms	800 mg Q 24 h	No Δ	600 mg Q 24 h	400 mg Q 24 h
Other					
Clindamycin	All indications/organisms	300 mg Q 6–8 h	No Δ	No Δ	No Δ
Fosfomycin	UTI/E. coli	3 g × 1	No Δ	No Δ	No Δ
Linezolid	All indications/organisms	600 mg Q 12 h	No Δ	No Δ	No Δ
Metronidazole	All indications/organisms	500 mg Q 8 h	No Δ	No Δ	No Δ
Nitrofurantoin	UTI/E. coli	100 mg Q 12 h	Not recommended	Not recommended	Not recommended
Rifampin	IE/MRSA (no monotherapy)	300 mg Q 8 h	No Δ	No Δ	No Δ
Trimethoprim/ sulfamethoxazole	SST/MRSA	2 DS tabs Q 12 h	No Δ	1 DS tab Q 12 h	Not recommended
	UTI/E. coli	1 DS tab Q 12 h	No Δ	1 SS tab Q 12 h	Not recommended
Vancomycin	CDI/Clostridium difficile	250 mg Q 6 h	No Δ	No Δ	No Δ

TABLE 2.1.5 Common Antimicrobial Adverse Effects and Monitoring

	Aminopenicillins	Nafcillin/oxacillin	PCN G	Piperacillin–tazobactam	Cefazolin	Cefepime	Ceftriaxone	Ertapenem	Imipenem/meropenem	Ciprofloxacin/levofloxacin	Moxifloxacin	Azithromycin	Doxycycline/minocycline	Amikacin	Gentamicin/tobramycin	Clindamycin	Daptomycin	Linezolid	Metronidazole	Tigecycline	Vancomycin
Daily neuro exam to monitor for neurotoxicity			X	X		X			X												
→ Altered mental status with excessive dosing			X	X		X															
→ Seizures with excessive dosing			X			X			X												
Tinnitus and/or hearing loss												X	X	X	X						
ECG at baseline and follow-up if necessary										X	X	X									
→ QTc interval if given with other QTc-prolonging drugs										X	X	X									
Diarrhea and/or GI upset	X		X	X				X	X	X	X	X	X			X			X[a]	X[b]	
Antibiotic-associated colitis/CDI										X	X					X					
ALT/AST/AlkP at baseline and weekly		X					X														
→ Acute cholestatic liver injury	X	X					X														
→ Acute hepatocellular necrosis	X	X																			

BUN/SCr at baseline and every 1–3 days

→ Acute kidney injury due to acute tubular necrosis

→ Acute kidney injury due to interstitial nephritis

→ Dose adjustment in reduced kidney function

May cause rash or anaphylaxis

Increased photosensitivity

CPK at baseline and every 3–7 days

CBC at baseline and every 1–3 days

→ Leukopenia

→ Thrombocytopenia

Therapeutic drug monitoring required

[a] Disulfuram reaction when given with EtOH.

[b] 10–20% risk of nausea and vomiting.

[c] May cause serotonin syndrome if given with other serotonergic drugs such as antidepressants, tramadol, opioids, triptans, CNS stimulants.

[d] Draw peak level 1 h after end of infusion of first dose (goal peak = 40–50) and 8–10 h random level (goal 8–10 h random <10).

[e] Draw peak level 1 h after end of infusion of first dose (goal peak = 20–25) and 8–10 h random level (goal 8–10 h random <5).

[f] Draw trough prior to 4th dose (goal trough 15–20 mg/L) (alternative goal trough 10–15 mg/L for SSTIs/IAIs).

TABLE 2.1.6 Susceptibility Breakpoint MIC (mg/L) Interpretive Criteria for Common Pathogens[a,b]

Class/Drugs	Enterobacteriaceae[c] CLSI	Enterobacteriaceae[c] EUCAST	Enterococcus spp. CLSI	Enterococcus spp. EUCAST	Pseudomonas Aeruginosa CLSI	Pseudomonas Aeruginosa EUCAST	Staphylococcus spp.[d] CLSI	Staphylococcus spp.[d] EUCAST	Streptococcus Pneumoniae CLSI	Streptococcus Pneumoniae EUCAST
PCNs										
Ampicillin	≤8	≤8	≤8				≤0.25		≤2	≤0.5
Amoxicillin	≤8	≤8						≤0.125	≤2	≤0.5
Ampicillin/sulbactam	≤8	≤8		≤4			≤8			≤0.5
Amoxicillin–clavulanate	≤8	≤8		≤4			≤4		≤2	≤0.5
Nafcillin							≤2			
Oxacillin (*S. aureus*)							≤2	≤2		
Oxacillin (*S. epidermidis*)							≤0.25	≤0.25		
PCN (non-CNS)[e]							≤0.125	≤0.125	≤2	≤2
PCN G (CNS)[f]									≤0.06	≤0.06
PCN VK									≤0.06	
Piperacillin–tazobactam[g]	≤16	≤8		≤4	≤16	≤16	≤8			
Cephalosporins										
Cefazolin	≤2									
Cefepime (non-CNS)[e]	≤8	≤1			≤8	≤8	≤8		≤1	≤1
Cefepime (CNS)[f]									≤0.5	≤0.5
Cefotaxime (non-CNS)[e]	≤1	≤1					≤8		≤1	≤0.5

Drug										
Cefotaxime (CNS)[f]	≤0.5									≤1
Ceftriaxone (non-CNS)[e]	≤1	≤1						≤8		≤1
Ceftriaxone (CNS)[f]	≤0.5	≤0.5								≤1
Carbapenems										
Ertapenem	≤0.5	≤0.5						≤2		≤1
Imipenem–cilastatin[g]	≤2	≤1			≤2	≤4		≤4		≤0.125
Meropenem[g]	≤2	≤1			≤2	≤2		≤4		≤0.25
Fluoroquinolones										
Ciprofloxacin[i,j]	≤1	≤0.5	≤1		≤1	≤0.5	≤1	≤1	≤1	≤1
Levofloxacin[i,j]	≤2	≤1	≤2		≤2	≤1	≤1	≤1	≤1	≤2
Moxifloxacin[j]	≤2	≤0.5			≤2		≤0.5	≤0.5	≤0.5	≤0.5
Macrolides										
Azithromycin[i]								≤2	≤1	≤0.25
Tetracyclines										
Doxycycline	≤4		≤4				≤4	≤4	≤1	≤1
Minocycline	≤4		≤4				≤4	≤4	≤0.5	≤0.5
Aminoglycosides[l]										≤0.5
Amikacin	≤16	≤8			≤16	≤8	≤8	≤16		
Gentamicin	≤4	≤2			≤4	≤4	≤1	≤1		≤1
Tobramycin	≤4	≤2			≤4	≤4	≤1	≤1		≤0.5

(Continued)

TABLE 2.1.6 Susceptibility Breakpoint MIC (mg/L) Interpretive Criteria for Common Pathogens[a,b] (Continued)

Class/Drugs	Enterobacteriaceae[c]		Pseudomonas Aeruginosa		Enterococcus spp.		Staphylococcus spp.[d]		Streptococcus Pneumoniae	
	CLSI	EUCAST	CLSI	EUCAST	CLSI	EUCAST	CLSI	EUCAST	CLSI	EUCAST
Other										
Clindamycin							≤0.5	≤0.25	≤0.25	≤0.5
Daptomycin					≤4		≤1	≤1		
Linezolid						≤4	≤4	≤4	≤2	≤2
Vancomycin[k]					≤4	≤4	≤2	≤2	≤1	≤2

[a] This table should NOT be used to compare potencies across antimicrobials. MIC breakpoints are drug-organism specific and antimicrobials have different PK properties.
[b] CLSI, EUCAST.
[c] Includes *Escherichia coli, Klebsiella* spp., *Proteus* spp., *Enterobacter, Citrobacter, Serratia*.
[d] If identified as MSSA, considered susceptible to amoxicillin–clavulanate, ampicillin–sulbactam, piperacillin–tazobactam, all cephalosporins and all carbapenems.
[e] Breakpoints applied to isolates *NOT* obtained from CSF in cases of CNS infections.
[f] Breakpoints applied to isolates obtained from CSF in cases of CNS infections.
[g] Penicillin-susceptible enterococci are also susceptible to imipenem, meropenem, and piperacillin—tazobactam.
[h] Meropenem susceptibility breakpoint for *S. pneumoniae* isolate obtained from CSF in cases of CNS infections is ≤0.25 mg/L.
[i] Ciprofloxacin and levofloxacin breakpoints should only be used for enterococci isolated from urine cultures.
[j] Not recommended as monotherapy for the treatment of serious *Staphylococcus* infections.
[k] Susceptibility breakpoint for coagulase-negative *Staphylococcus* is ≤4 mg/L.

FIGURE 2.2.1 Osteomyelitis

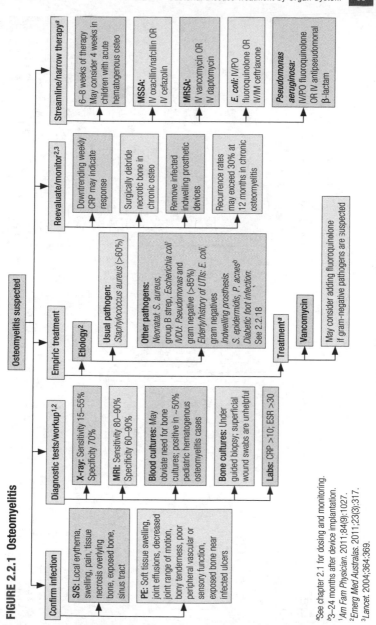

[a]See chapter 2.1 for dosing and monitoring.
[b]3–24 months after device implantation.
[1]Am Fam Physician. 2011;84(9):1027.
[2]Emerg Med Australas. 2011;23(3):317.
[3]Lancet. 2004;364:369.

FIGURE 2.2.2 Septic Arthritis

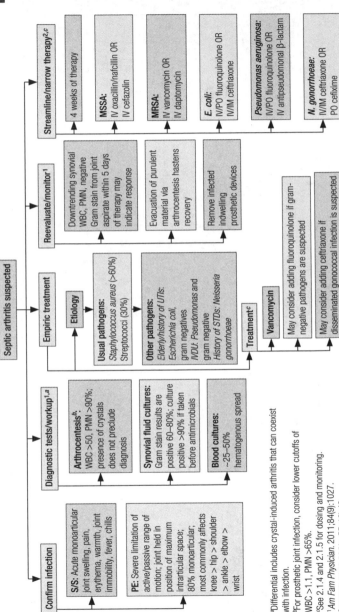

Confirm infection

S/S: Acute monoarticular joint swelling, pain, erythema, warmth, joint immobility, fever, chills

PE: Severe limitation of active/passive range of motion; joint held in position of maximum intrarticular space; 80% monoarticular; most commonly affects knee > hip > shoulder > ankle > elbow > wrist

Diagnostic tests/workup[1,a]

Arthrocentesis[b]: WBC >50, PMN >90%; presence of crystals does not preclude diagnosis

Synovial fluid cultures: Gram stain results are positive 60–80%; culture positive >90% if taken before antimicrobials

Blood cultures: ~25–50% hematogenous spread

Empiric treatment

Etiology

Usual pathogens: *Staphylococcus aureus* (>60%) Streptococci (30%)

Other pathogens: *Elderly/history of UTIs:* *Escherichia coli,* gram negatives *IVDU:* Pseudomonas and gram negative *History of STDS: Neisseria gonorrhoeae*

Treatment[c]

Vancomycin

May consider adding fluoroquinolone if gram-negative pathogens are suspected

May consider adding ceftriaxone if disseminated gonococcal infection is suspected

Reevaluate/monitor[1]

Downtrending synovial WBC, PMN, negative Gram stain from joint aspirate within 5 days of therapy may indicate response

Evacuation of purulent material via arthrocentesis hastens recovery

Remove infected indwelling prosthetic devices

Streamline/narrow therapy[2,c]

4 weeks of therapy

MSSA: IV oxacillin/nafcillin OR IV cefazolin

MRSA: IV vancomycin OR IV daptomycin

E. coli: IV/PO fluoroquinolone OR IV/IM ceftriaxone

Pseudomonas aeruginosa: IV/PO fluoroquinolone OR IV antipseudomonal β-lactam

N. gonorrhoeae: IV/IM ceftriaxone OR PO cefixime

Septic arthritis suspected

[a]Differential includes crystal-induced arthritis that can coexist with infection.
[b]For prosthetic joint infection, consider lower cutoffs of WBC >1.1, PMN >65%.
[c]See 2.1.4 and 2.1.5 for dosing and monitoring.
[1]*Am Fam Physician.* 2011;84(9):1027.
[2]*MMWR.* 2010;59(No. RR-12):49.

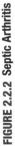

FIGURE 2.2.3 Catheter-Related Bloodstream Infections

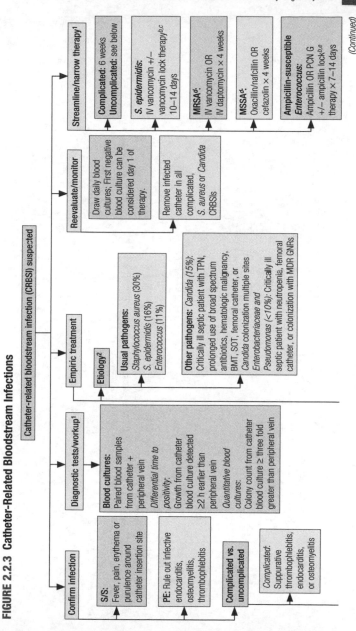

(Continued)

FIGURE 2.2.3 Catheter-Related Bloodstream Infections (*Continued*)

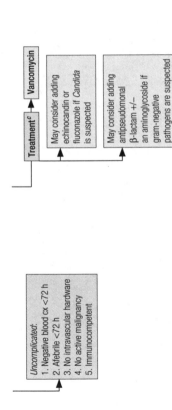

Uncomplicated:
1. Negative blood cx <72 h
2. Afebrile <72 r
3. No intravascular hardware
4. No active malignancy
5. Immunocompetent

Treatment[c] → Vancomycin

May consider adding echinocandin or fluconazole if *Candida* is suspected

May consider adding antipseudomonal β-lactam +/− an aminoglycoside if gram-negative pathogens are suspected

[a]See chapter 2.1 for dosing and monitoring.
[b]If uncomplicated with long-term catheter, may salvage catheter by giving systemic + antibiotic lock therapy.
[c]Vancomycin 5 mg/mL +/− heparin 5,000 units/mL with catheter dwell times 24–48 h.
[d]May use 2 weeks for *S. aureus* only if patient meets all criteria for uncomplicated and does not have diabetes.
[e]Ampicillin 10 mg/mL +/− heparin 5,000 units/mL with catheter dwell times 24–48 h.
[1]*Clin Infect Dis.* 2009;49:1.
[2]*Am J Med.* 2010;123(9):819.

FIGURE 2.2.4 Infective Endocarditis

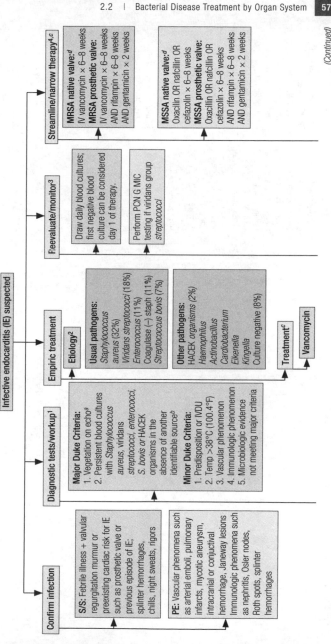

(Continued)

FIGURE 2.2.4 Infective Endocarditis *(Continued)*

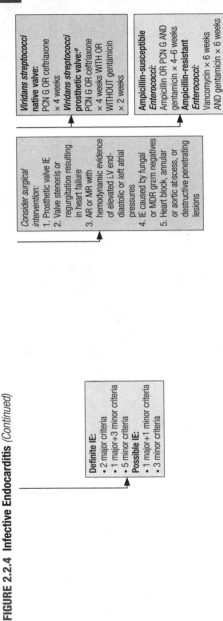

Viridans streptococci native valve:
PCN G OR ceftriaxone × 4 weeks
Viridans streptococci prosthetic valve:[e]
PCN G OR ceftriaxone × 4 weeks WITH OR WITHOUT gentamicin × 2 weeks

Ampicillin-susceptible *Enterococci:*
Ampicillin OR PCN G AND gentamicin × 4–6 weeks
Ampicillin-resistant *Enterococci:*
Vancomycin × 6 weeks AND gentamicin × 6 weeks

Consider surgical intervention:
1. Prosthetic valve IE
2. Valve stenosis or regurgitation resulting in heart failure
3. AR or MR with hemodynamic evidence of elevated LV end-diastolic or left atrial pressures
4. IE caused by fungal or MDR gram negatives
5. Heart block, annular or aortic abscess, or destructive penetrating lesions

Definite IE:
• 2 major criteria
• 1 major+3 minor criteria
• 5 minor criteria
Possible IE:
• 1 major+1 minor criteria
• 3 minor criteria

[a]Oscillating intracardiac mass on valve, abscess, or new partial dehiscence of prosthetic valve.
[b]Two blood cultures drawn >12 h apart or 3 of 4 positive blood cultures drawn >1 h apart
[c]See chapter 2.1 for dosing and monitoring.
[d]Daptomycin is noninferior to therapy for right-sided IE (*N Engl J Med* 2006;355:653).
[e]If PCN MIC ≥0.25 → Duration is 6 weeks of β-lactam AND gentamicin.

[1] *Clin Infect Dis.* 2000;30:633.
[2] *JAMA.* 2005;293:3012.
[3] *J Am Coll Cardiol.* 2008;52:1.
[4] *Circulation* 2005;111:e394.

FIGURE 2.2.5 *Clostridium difficile* Infection

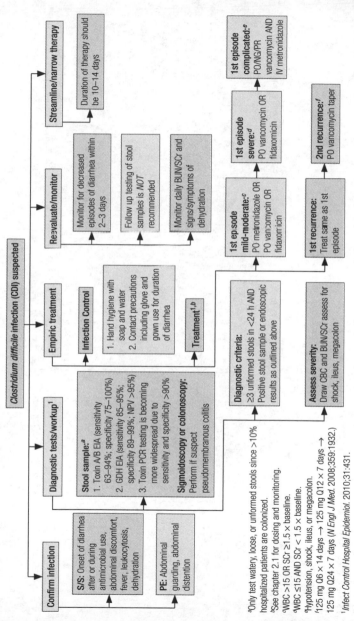

Clostridium difficile infection (CDI) suspected

Confirm infection

S/S: Onset of diarrhea after or during antimicrobial use, abdominal discomfort, fever, leukocytosis, dehydration

PE: Abdominal guarding, abdominal distention

Diagnostic tests/workup[1]

Stool sample:[a]
1. Toxin A/B EIA (sensitivity 63–94%, specificity 75–100%)
2. GDH EIA (sensitivity 85–95%; specificity 89–99%; NPV >95%)
3. Toxin PCR testing is becoming more widespread due to sensitivity and specificity >90%

Sigmoidoscopy or colonoscopy: Perform if suspect pseudomembranous colitis

Empiric treatment

Infection Control
1. Hand hygiene with soap and water
2. Contact precautions including glove and gown use for duration of diarrhea

Treatment[1,b]

Diagnostic criteria:
≥3 unformed stools in <24 h AND Positive stool sample or endoscopic results as outlined above

Assess severity:
Draw CBC and BUN/SCr assess for shock, ileus, megacolon

Re-evaluate/monitor

Monitor for decreased episodes of diarrhea within 2–3 days

Follow up testing of stool samples is *NOT* recommended

Monitor daily BUN/SCr and signs/symptoms of dehydration

Streamline/narrow therapy

Duration of therapy should be 10–14 days

1st episode mild–moderate:[c]
PO metronidazole OR PO vancomycin OR fidaxomicin

1st episode severe:[d]
PO vancomycin OR fidaxomicin

1st episode complicated:[e]
PO/NG/PR vancomycin AND IV metronidazole

1st recurrence:
Treat same as 1st episode

2nd recurrence:[f]
PO vancomycin taper

[a]Only test watery, loose, or unformed stools since >10% hospitalized patients are colonized.
[b]See chapter 2.1 for dosing and monitoring.
[c]WBC >15 OR SCr ≥1.5 × baseline.
[d]WBC ≤15 AND SCr < 1.5 × baseline.
[e]Hypotension, shock, ileus, or megacolon.
[f]125 mg Q6 × 14 days → 125 mg Q12 × 7 days → 125 mg Q24 × 7 days (*N Engl J Med.* 2008;359:1932.)
[1]*Infect Control Hospital Epidemiol.* 2010;31:431.

FIGURE 2.2.6 Intra-Abdominal Infections

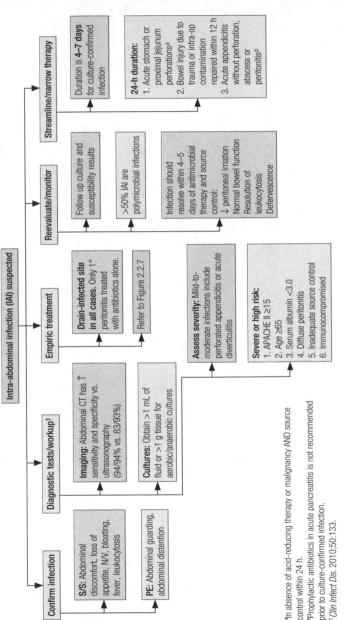

Confirm infection

S/S: Abdominal discomfort, loss of appetite, N/V, bloating, fever, leukocytosis

PE: Abdominal guarding, abdominal distention

Diagnostic tests/workup[1]

Imaging: Abdominal CT has ↑ sensitivity and specificity vs. ultrasonography (94/94% vs. 83/93%)

Cultures: Obtain >1 mL of fluid or >1 g tissue for aerobic/anaerobic cultures

Intra-abdominal infection (IAI) suspected

Empiric treatment

Drain-infected site in all cases. Only 1° peritonitis treated with antibiotics alone.

Refer to Figure 2.2.7

Assess severity: Mild-to-moderate infections include perforated appendicitis or acute diverticulitis

Severe or high risk:
1. APACHE II ≥15
2. Age ≥65
3. Serum albumin <3.0
4. Diffuse peritonitis
5. Inadequate source control
6. Immunocompromised

Reevaluate/monitor

Follow up culture and susceptibility results

>50% IAI are polymicrobial infections

Infection should resolve within 4–5 days of antimicrobial therapy and source control:
↓ peritoneal irriation
Normal bowel function
Resolution of leukocytosis
Defervescence

Streamline/narrow therapy

Duration is **4–7 days** for culture-confirmed infection

24-h duration:
1. Acute stomach or proximal jejunum perforations[a]
2. Bowel injury due to trauma or intra-op contamination repaired within 12 h
3. Acute appendicitis without perforation, abscess or peritonitis[b]

[a]In absence of acid-reducing therapy or malignancy AND source control within 24 h.
[b]Prophylactic antibiotics in acute pancreatitis is not recommended prior to culture-confirmed infection.
[1]*Clin Infect Dis.* 2010;50:133.

FIGURE 2.2.7 Empiric Therapy for IAI

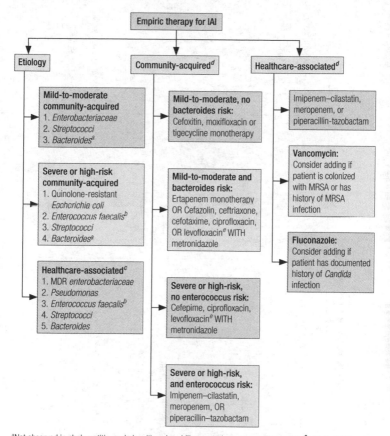

[a]Not observed in cholecystitis or cholangitis unless biliary-enteric anastomosis present; ↑ risk in distal small bowel, appendiceal, colonic, paralytic ileus, or proximal GI perforations with obstruction.

[b]Not pathogenic in biliary infections; ↑ risk with post-op infection, previous receipt of cephalosporins, immunocompromised, valvular heart diseases, or intravascular devices.

[c]Presence of invasive device, history of surgery, hospitalization, residence in long-term care facility, or dialysis within 12 months, onset >48 h of hospital admission.

[d]See chapter 2.1 for dosing and monitoring.

[e]Fluoroquinolones should only be used if antibiogram shows >90% susceptibility to E. coli.

FIGURE 2.2.8 Acute Bacterial Meningitis

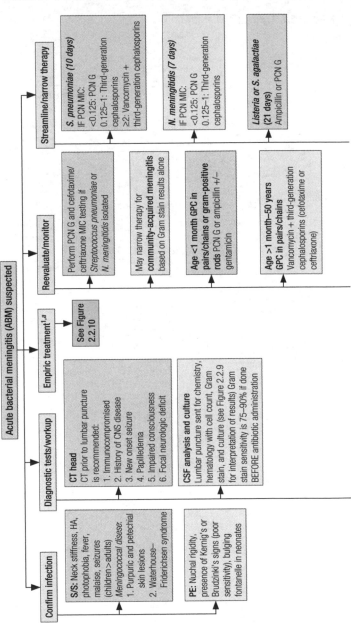

Acute bacterial meningitis (ABM) suspected

Confirm infection

S/S: Neck stiffness, HA, photophobia, fever, malaise, seizures
Meningococcal disease:
1. Purpuric and petechial skin lesions
2. Waterhouse–Friderichsen syndrome
Meningococcal disease (children >adults)

PE: Nuchal rigidity, presence of Kernig's or Brudzinki's signs (poor sensitivity), bulging fontanelle in neonates

Diagnostic tests/workup

CT head
CT prior to lumbar puncture is recommended:
1. Immunocompromised
2. History of CNS disease
3. New onset seizure
4. Papilledema
5. Impaired consciousness
6. Focal neurologic deficit

CSF analysis and culture
Lumbar puncture sent for chemistry, hematology with cell count, Gram stain, and culture (see Figure 2.2.9 for interpretation of results) Gram stain sensitivity is 75–90% if done BEFORE antibiotic administration

Empiric treatment[1,a]

See Figure 2.2.10

Reevaluate/monitor

Perform PCN G and cefotaxime/ceftriaxone MIC testing if *Streptococcus pneumoniae* or *N. meningitidis* isolated

May narrow therapy for **community-acquired meningitis** based on Gram stain results alone

Age <1 month GPC in pairs/chains or gram-positive rods PCN G or ampicillin +/– gentamicin

Age >1 month–50 years GPC in pairs/chains Vancomycin + third-generation cephalosporins (cefotaxime or ceftriaxone)

Streamline/narrow therapy

S. pneumoniae (10 days)
IF PCN MIC:
<0.125: PCN G
0.125–1: Third-generation cephalosporins
≥2: Vancomycin + third-generation cephalosporins

N. meningitidis (7 days)
IF PCN MIC:
<0.125: PCN G
0.125–1: Third-generation cephalosporins

Listeria or *S. agalactiae* (21 days)
Ampicillin or PCN G

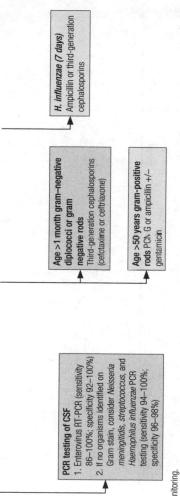

H. influenzae (7 days)
Ampicillin or third-generation cephalosporins

Age >1 month gram-negative diplococci or gram negative rods
Third-generation cephalosporins (cefotaxime or ceftriaxone)

Age >50 years gram-positive rods PCN G or ampicillin +/− gentamicin

PCR testing of CSF
1. Enterovirus RT-PCR (sensitivity 86–100%; specificity 92–100%)
2. If no organisms identified on Gram stain, consider *Neisseria meningitidis, streptococcus,* and *Haemophilus influenzae* PCR testing (sensitivity 94–100%; specificity 96–98%)

ᵃSee chapter 2.1 for dosing and monitoring.
¹*Clin Infect Dis.* 2004;39:1267.

TABLE 2.2.9 Cerebrospinal Fluid Analysis

	Normal	Bacterial	Viral	Fungal	TB
WBC	<5	1,000–5,000	100–1,000	40–400	100–500
Diff%	>90 monos	≥80 PMNs	50 lymphs	>50 lymphs	>80 lymphs
Protein	<50	100–500	30–150	40–150	<40–150
Glucose	50–60% of blood glucose	<60% of blood glucose	<30–70	<30–70	<30–70

FIGURE 2.2.10 Empiric Therapy for ABM

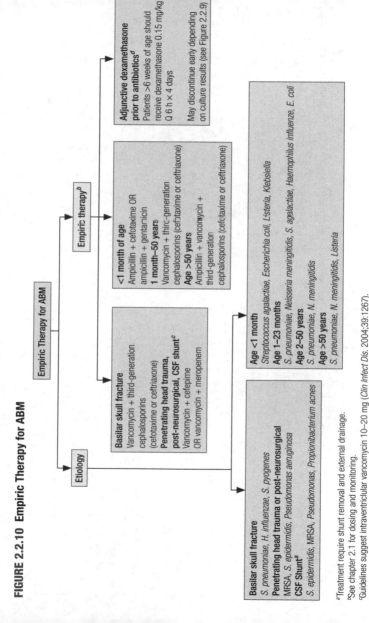

Empiric Therapy for ABM

Etiology

Empiric therapy[b]

Basilar skull fracture
Vancomycin + third-generation cephalosporins (cefotaxime or ceftriaxone)
Penetrating head trauma, post-neurosurgical, CSF shunt[c]
Vancomycin + cefepime
OR vancomycin + meropenem

<1 month of age
Ampicillin + cefotaxime OR ampicillin + gentamicin
1 month–50 years
Vancomycin + third-generation cephalosporins (cefotaxime or ceftriaxone)
Age >50 years
Ampicillin + vancomycin + third-generation cephalosporins (cefotaxime or ceftriaxone)

Adjunctive dexamethasone prior to antibiotics[d]
Patients >6 weeks of age should receive dexamethasone 0.15 mg/kg
Q 6 h × 4 days
May discontinue early depending on culture results (see Figure 2.2.9)

Basilar skull fracture
S. pneumoniae, H. influenzae, S. pyogenes
Penetrating head trauma or post-neurosurgical
MRSA, S. epidermidis, Pseudomonas aeruginosa
CSF Shunt[a]
S. epidermidis, MRSA, Pseudomonas, Propionibacterium acnes

Age <1 month
Streptococcus agalactiae, Escherichia coli, Listeria, Klebsiella
Age 1–23 months
S. pneumoniae, Neisseria meningitidis, S. agalactiae, Haemophilus influenze, E. coli
Age 2–50 years
S. pneumoniae, N. meningitidis
Age >50 years
S. pneumoniae, N. meningitidis, Listeria

[a]Treatment require shunt removal and external drainage.
[b]See chapter 2.1 for dosing and monitoring.
[c]Guidelines suggest intraventricular vancomycin 10–20 mg (Clin Infect Dis. 2004;39:1267).
[d]Can be used without affecting vancomycin CSF concentration (Clin Infect Dis. 2007;44:250).

FIGURE 2.2.11 Acute Otitis Media

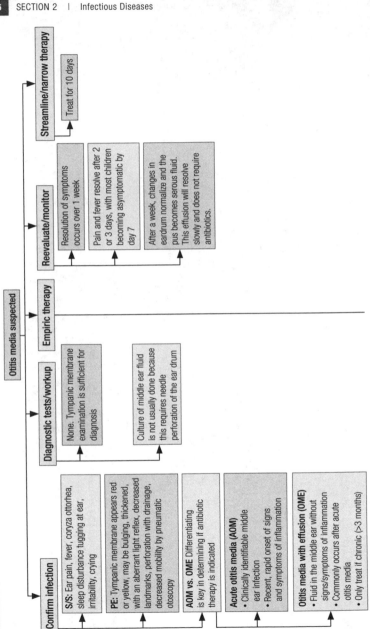

Otitis media suspected

Confirm infection

S/S: Ear pain, fever, coryza ottorhea, sleep disturbance tugging at ear, irritability, crying

PE: Tympanic membrane appears red or yellow, may be bulging, thickened, with an aberrant light reflex, decreased landmarks, perforation with drainage, decreased mobility by pneumatic otoscopy

AOM vs. OME Differentiating is key in determining if antibiotic therapy is indicated

Acute otitis media (AOM)
• Clinically identifiable middle ear infection
• Recent, rapid onset of signs and symptoms of inflammation

Otitis media with effusion (OME)
• Fluid in the middle ear without signs/symptoms of inflammation
• Commonly occurs after acute otitis media
• Only treat if chronic (>3 months)

Diagnostic tests/workup

None. Tympanic membrane examination is sufficient for diagnosis

Culture of middle ear fluid is not usually done because this requires needle perforation of the ear drum

Empiric therapy

Reevaluate/monitor

Resolution of symptoms occurs over 1 week

Pain and fever resolve after 2 or 3 days, with most children becoming asymptomatic by day 7

After a week, changes in eardrum normalize and the pus becomes serous fluid. This effusion will resolve slowly and does not require antibiotics.

Streamline/narrow therapy

Treat for 10 days

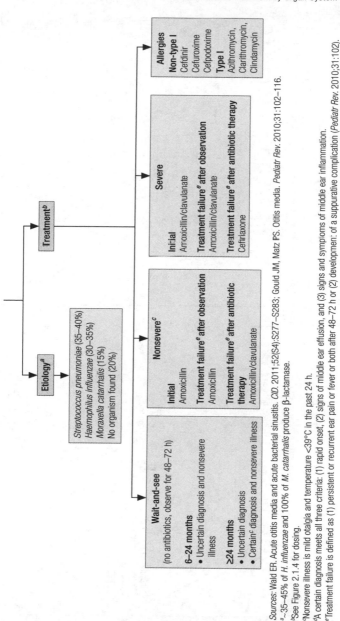

Etiology[a]

Streptococcus pneumoniae (35–40%)
Haemophilus influenzae (30–35%)
Moraxella catarrhalis (15%)
No organism found (20%)

Treatment[b]

Wait-and-see
(no antibiotics, observe for 48–72 h)

6–24 months
• Uncertain diagnosis and nonsevere illness

≥24 months
• Uncertain diagnosis
• Certain[c] diagnosis and nonsevere illness

Nonsevere[c]

Initial
Amoxicillin

Treatment failure[e] **after observation**
Amoxicillin

Treatment failure[e] **after antibiotic therapy**
Amoxicillin/clavulanate

Severe

Initial
Amoxicillin/clavulanate

Treatment failure[e] **after observation**
Amoxicillin/clavulanate

Treatment failure[e] **after antibiotic therapy**
Ceftriaxone

Allergies
Non-type I
Cefdinir
Cefuroxime
Cefpodoxime
Type I
Azithromycin,
Clarithromycin,
Clindamycin

Sources: Wald ER. Acute otitis media and acute bacterial sinusitis. *CID.* 2011;52(S4):S277–S283; Gould JM, Matz PS. Otitis media. *Pediatr Rev.* 2010;31:102–116.
[a] 35–45% of *H. influenzae* and 100% of *M. catarrhalis* produce β-lactamase.
[b] See Figure 2.1.4 for dosing.
[c] Nonsevere illness is mild otalgia and temperature <39°C in the past 24 h.
[d] A certain diagnosis meets all three criteria: (1) rapid onset; (2) signs of middle ear effusion, and (3) signs and symptoms of middle ear inflammation.
[e] Treatment failure is defined as (1) persistent or recurrent ear pain or fever or both after 48–72 h or (2) development of a suppurative complication (*Pediatr Rev.* 2010;31:102).

FIGURE 2.2.12 Pharyngitis

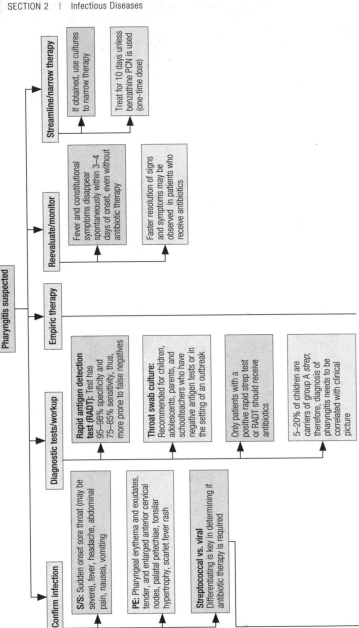

Pharyngitis suspected

Confirm infection

S/S: Sudden onset sore throat (may be severe), fever, headache, abdominal pain, nausea, vomiting

PE: Pharyngeal erythema and exudates, tender, and enlarged anterior cervical nodes, palatal petechiae, tonsilar hypertrophy, scarlet fever rash

Streptococcal vs. viral
Differentiating is key in determining if antibiotic therapy is required

Diagnostic tests/workup

Rapid antigen detection test (RADT): Test has 95–98% specificity and 75–85% sensitivity; thus, more prone to false negatives

Throat swab culture: Recommended for children, adolescents, parents, and schoolteachers who have negative antigen tests or in the setting of an outbreak

Only patients with a positive rapid strep test or RADT should receive antibiotics

5–20% of children are carriers of group A *strep*, therefore, diagnosis of pharyngitis needs to be correlated with clinical picture

Empiric therapy

Reevaluate/monitor

Fever and constitutional symptoms disappear spontaneously within 3–4 days of onset, even without antibiotic therapy

Faster resolution of signs and symptoms may be observed in patients who receive antibiotics

Streamline/narrow therapy

If obtained, use cultures to narrow therapy

Treat for 10 days unless benzathine PCN is used (one-time dose)

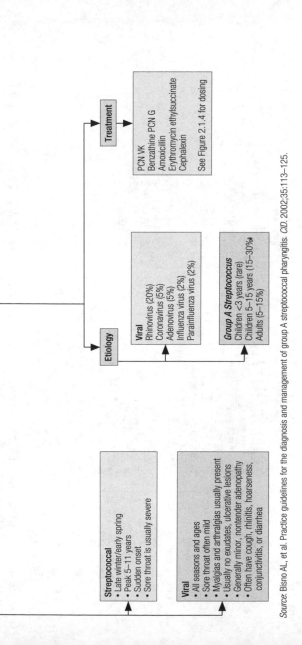

Streptococcal
- Late winter/early spring
- Peak 5–11 years
- Sudden onset
- Sore throat is usually severe

Viral
- All seasons and ages
- Sore throat often mild
- Myalgias and arthralgias usually present
- Usually no exudates, ulcerative lesions
- Generally minor, nontender adenopathy
- Often have cough, rhinitis, hoarseness, conjunctivitis, or diarrhea

Etiology

Viral
Rhinovirus (20%)
Coronavirus (5%)
Adenovirus (5%)
Influenza virus (2%)
Parainfluenza virus (2%)

Group A Streptococcus
Children <3 years (rare)
Children 5–15 years (15–30%)
Adults (5–15%)

Treatment

PCN VK
Benzathine PCN G
Amoxicillin
Erythromycin ethylsuccinate
Cephalexin

See Figure 2.1.4 for dosing

Source: Bisno AL, et al: Practice guidelines for the diagnosis and management of group A streptococcal pharyngitis. *CID.* 2002;35:113–125.

FIGURE 2.2.13 Community-Acquired Pneumonia

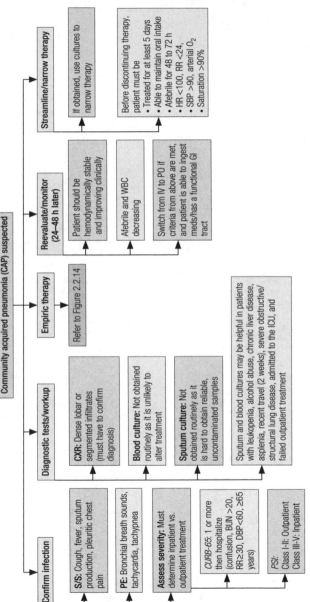

Source: Mandell LA, Wunderink RG, Anzueto A, Bartlett JG, Campbell GD, et al. Infectious Diseases Society of America /American Thoracic Society consensus guidelines on the management of community-acquired pneumonia. *CID* 2007;44:S27–S72.

FIGURE 2.2.14 Empiric Therapy for CAP

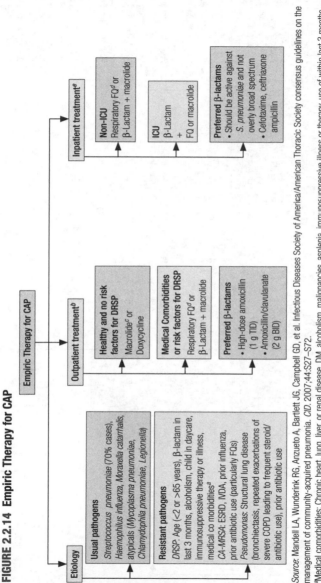

Source: Mandell LA, Wunderink RG, Anzueto A, Bartlett JG, Campbell GD, et al. Infectious Diseases Society of America/American Thoracic Society consensus guidelines on the management of community-acquired pneumonia. *CID.* 2007;44:S27–S72.

[a]Medical comorbidities: Chronic heart, lung, liver, or renal disease, DM, alcoholism, malignancies, asplenia, immunosuppressive illness or therapy, use of within last 3 months.

[b]See figure 2.1.4 for dosing.

[c]Do not use macrolide monotherapy if >25% high level (MIC ≥16) macrolide resistance to *S. penumoniae.*

[d]Respiratory FQ: levofloxacin, moxifloxacin, gemifloxacin.

[e]See figures 2.1.2 and 2.1.3 for dosing.

FIGURE 2.2.15 Hospital-Acquired Pneumonia/Ventilator-Associated Pneumonia

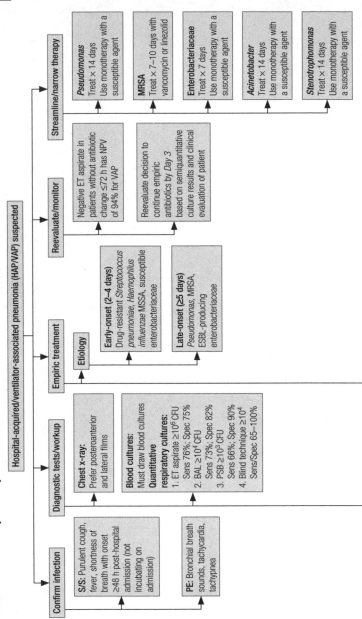

Hospital-acquired/ventilator-associated pneumonia (HAP/VAP) suspected

Confirm infection

S/S: Purulent cough, fever, shortness of breath with onset ≥48 h post-hospital admission (not incubating on admission)

PE: Bronchial breath sounds, tachycardia, tachypnea

Diagnostic tests/workup

Chest x-ray: Prefer posteroanterior and lateral films

Blood cultures: Must draw blood cultures
Quantitative respiratory cultures:
1. ET aspirate ≥10⁶ CFU Sens 76%; Spec 75%
2. BAL ≥10⁴ CFU Sens 73%; Spec 82%
3. PSB ≥10³ CFU Sens 66%; Spec 90%
4. Blind technique ≥10⁴ Sens/Spec 65–100%

Empiric treatment

Etiology

Early-onset (2–4 days) Drug-resistant *Streptococcus pneumoniae*, *Haemophilus influenzae* MSSA, susceptible enterobacteriaceae

Late-onset (≥5 days) *Pseudomonas*, MRSA, ESBL-producing enterobacteriaceae

Reevaluate/monitor

Negative ET aspirate in patients without antibiotic change ≤72 h has NPV of 94% for VAP

Reevaluate decision to continue empiric antibiotics by *Day 3* based on semiquantitative culture results and clinical evaluation of patient

Streamline/narrow therapy

Pseudomonas Treat × 14 days Use monotherapy with a susceptible agent

MRSA Treat × 7–10 days with vancomycin or linezolid

Enterobacteriaceae Treat × 7 days Use monotherapy with a susceptible agent

Acinetobacter Treat × 14 days Use monotherapy with a susceptible agent

Stenotrophomonas Treat × 14 days Use monotherapy with a susceptible agent

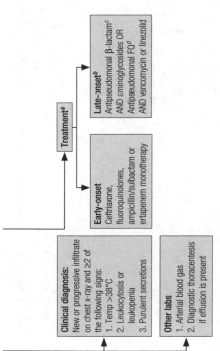

Clinical diagnosis:
New or progressive infiltrate on chest x-ray and ≥2 of the following signs:
1. Temp >38°C
2. Leukocytosis or leukopenia
3. Purulent secretions

Other labs
1. Arterial blood gas
2. Diagnostic thoracentesis if effusion is present

Treatment[a]

Early-onset
Ceftriaxone, fluoroquinolones, ampicillin/sulbactam or ertapenem monotherapy

Late-onset[b]
Antipseudomonal β-lactam[c] AND aminoglycosides OR Antipseudomonal FQ[d] AND vancomycin or linezolid

[a]See chapter 2.1 for dosing and monitoring.
[b]Strongly consider two antipseudomonal agents if local susceptibility to one drug is <90% and patient critically ill.
[c]Imipenem-cilastatin, meropenem, doripenem.
[d]Ciprofloxacin or levofloxacin.

FIGURE 2.2.16 Abscesses and Cellulitis

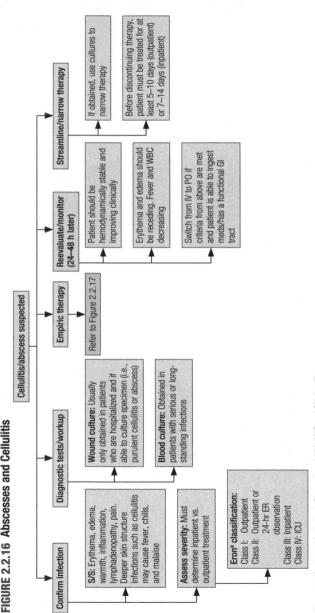

aEron classification (J Antimicrob Chemother. 2003;52(Suppl S1):3–17).
Class I: Afebrile and healthy, other than cellulitis.
Class II: Febrile and ill-appearing, but no unstable comorbidities (PVD, DM, antibiotic use in the last 2 weeks, alcohol abuse, advanced age, chronic liver and/or renal disease, asplenia).
Class III: Toxic appearance, or at least one unstable comorbidity, or a limb-threatening infection.
Class IV: Sepsis syndrome or life-threatening infection (i.e., necrotizing fasciitis).

FIGURE 2.2.17 Empiric Therapy for Abscesses and Cellulitis

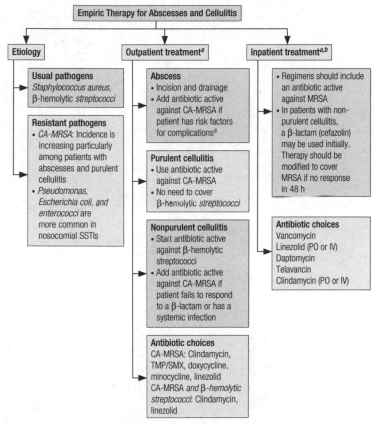

Sources: (1) Eron LJ, et al. Managing skin and soft tissue infections: expert panel recommendations on key decision points. *J Antimicrob Chemother*. 2003;52:S1:i3–i17; (2) Stevens DL, et al. Practice guidelines for the diagnosis and management of skin and soft tissue infections. *CID*. 2005;41:1373–1406; (3) Liu C, Bayer A, Cosgrove SE, Daum RS, Fridkin SK, et al. Clinical practice guidelines by the Infectious Diseases Society of America for the treatment of methicillin-resistant Staphylococcus aureus infections in adults and children. *CID*. 2011;52(1):1.

[a]See chapter 2.1 for dosing and monitoring.

[b]Severe or extensive disease (e.g., involving multiple sites of infection) or rapid progression in presence of associated cellulitis, signs and symptoms of systemic illness, associated comorbidities or immunosuppression, extremes of age, abscess in an area difficult to drain (e.g., face, hand, and genitalia), associated septic phlebitis, and lack of response to incision and drainage.

FIGURE 2.2.18 Diabetic Foot Ulcers

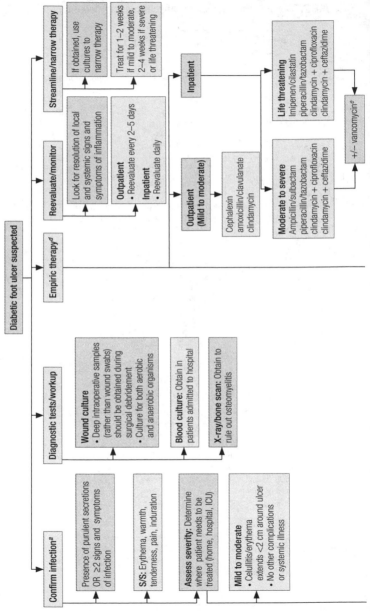

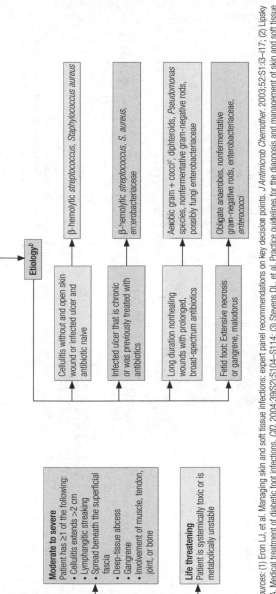

Moderate to severe

Patient has ≥1 of the following:
- Cellulitis extends >2 cm
- Lymphangitic streaking
- Spread beneath the superficial fascia
- Deep-tissue abcess
- Gangrene
- Involvement of muscle, tendon, joint, or bone

Life threatening

Patient is systemically toxic or is metabolically unstable

Etiology[b]

Cellulitis without and open skin wound or infected ulcer and antibiotic naive	β-hemolytic *streptococcus*, *Staphylococcus aureus*
Infected ulcer that is chronic or was previously treated with antibiotics	β-hemolytic *streptococcus*, *S. aureus*, enterobacteriaceae
Long duration nonhealing wounds with prolonged, broad-spectrum antibiotics	Aerobic gram + cocci[c], diphtheroids, *Pseudomonas* species, nonfermentative gram-negative rods, possibly fungi enterobacteriaceae
Fetid foot: Extensive necrosis or gangrene, malodorus	Obligate anaerobes, nonfermentative gram-negative rods, enterobacteriaceae, *enterococci*

Sources: (1) Eron LJ, et al. Managing skin and soft tissue infections: expert panel recommendations on key decision points. *J Antimicrob Chemother.* 2003;52:S1:i3–i17; (2) Lipsky BA. Medical treatment of diabetic foot infections. *CID.* 2004;39(S2):S104–S114; (3) Stevens DL, et al. Practice guidelines for the diagnosis and management of skin and soft tissue infections. *CID.* 2005;41:1373–1406; (4) Lipsky BA, et al. Diagnosis and treatment of diabetic foot infections. *CID.* 2004;39:885–910; (5) Liu C, Bayer A, Cosgrove SE, Daum RS, Fridkin SK, et al. Clinical practice guidelines by the Infectious Diseases Society of America for the treatment of methicillin-resistant Staphylococcus aureus infections in adults and children. *CID.* 2011;52(1):1–38.

[b]Diagnosis cannot be made based on microbiological results as most open wounds are colonized.
[b]Pseudomonas is usually found in ulcers that are macerated because of soaking.
[c]Aerobic gram-positive: cocci: *S. aureus*, coagulase-negative *staphylococci*, *enterococci*.
[d]See chapter 2.1 for dosing and monitoring.
[e]Consider using vancomycin if high rates of methicillin-resistant *S. aureus* are found in the hospital or community.

FIGURE 2.2.19 Urinary Tract Infections

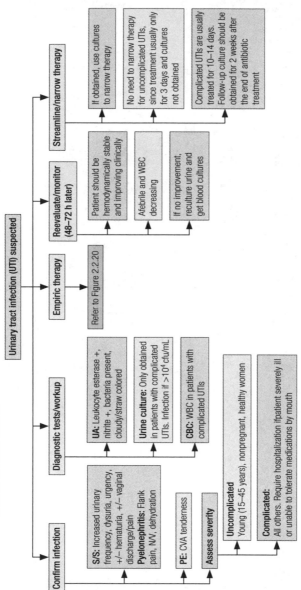

Source: (1) Drekonja DM, et al. Urinary tract infections. *Prim Care Clin Office Pract.* 2008;35:345–367; (2) Simerville JA, et al. Urinalysis: A comprehensive review. *Am Fam Physician.* 2005;71:1153–1162; (3) Gupta K, Hooton TM, Naber KG, Wullt B, Colgan R, et al. International clinical practice guidelines for the treatment of acute uncomplicated cystitis and pyelonephritis in women: A 2010 update by the Infectious Diseases Society of America and the European Society for Microbiology and Infectious Diseases. *CID.* 2011;52(5):e103–e120.

FIGURE 2.2.20 Empiric Therapy for UTIs

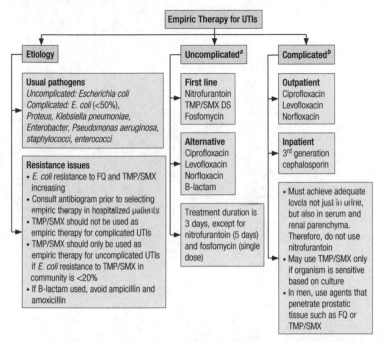

Sources: (1) Drekonja DM, et al. Urinary tract infections. *Prim Care Clin Office Pract.* 2008;35:345–367; (2) Simerville JA, et al. Urinalysis: A comprehensive review. *Am Fam Physician.* 2005;71:1153–1162; (3) Gupta K, Hooton TM, Naber KG, Wullt B, Colgan R, et al. International clinical practice guidelines for the treatment of acute uncomplicated cystitis and pyelonephritis in women: A 2010 update by the Infectious Diseases Society of America and the European Society for Microbiology and Infectious Diseases. *CID.* 2011;52(5):e103–e120.

[a]See chapter 2.1 for dosing and monitoring.

[b]UTIs are considered complicated if they occur in men, the elderly (>65 years), include sites other than the bladder, or the patient has "predisposing factors". Such factors include diabetes, congenital abnormalities of the urinary tract, a stone, indwelling catheter, prostatic hypertrophy, obstruction, or neurologic deficit that interfere with the normal flow of urine or voiding mechanism.

TABLE 2.3.1 Antifungal Formulations and Dosing

Drug	Brand Name	Available Formulations	General Dose Range
Azoles			
Fluconazole	Diflucan	Oral (tablets and suspension)	100–800 mg once daily
		Intravenous	(6–12 mg/kg/day for systemic infections)
Itraconazole	Sporanox	Capsules and oral solution (solution contains cyclodextrin)	200 mg QD to three times daily[a,b]
Posaconazole	Noxafil	Oral suspension	200 mg three to four times daily
			400 mg once to twice daily[c]
Voriconazole	Vfend	Oral (tablet and suspension)	6 mg/kg IV every 12 h for 24 h, then 4 mg/kg IV (200–300 mg PO) every 12 h[d]
		Intravenous (IV formulation contains cyclodextrin)	
Echinocandins			
Anidulafungin	Eraxis	Intravenous	Invasive candidiasis—200 mg IV on day 1, then 100 mg IV every 24 h
			Esophageal candidiasis—100 mg IV on day 1, then 50 mg IV every 24 h
Caspofungin	Cancidas	Intravenous	70 mg IV on day 1, then 50 mg IV every 24 h
Micafungin	Mycamine	Intravenous	Invasive candidiasis—100–150 mg IV every 24 h
			Esophageal candidiasis—150 mg IV every 24 h
			Prophylaxis—50 mg IV every 24 h

Polyenes			
Amphotericin B deoxycholate	Fungizone	Intravenous	0.5–1.0 mg/kg IV every 24 h
Amphotericin B colloidal dispersion	Amphotec (ABCD)	Intravenous	3–5 mg/kg IV every 24 h
Amphotericin B lipid complex	Abelcet (ABLC)	Intravenous	3–5 mg/kg IV every 24 h
Liposomal amphotericin B	Ambisome (LAMB)	Intravenous	3–5 mg/kg IV every 24 h
Miscellaneous			
Flucytosine	Ancobon	Oral (capsules)	25 mg/kg PO every 6 h
Terbinafine	Lamisil	Oral (granules and tablets)	250 mg PO once daily

[a]Administer oral solution on empty stomach.
[b]Administer capsules with food.
[c]Administer with food (preferably a fatty meal).
[d]Administer tablets and suspension on empty stomach.

TABLE 2.3.2 Antifungal Adverse Effects

Agent	Adverse Effects
Azoles[a]	
Fluconazole	Generally well-tolerated; increases in liver function tests and possibility of hepatotoxicity (class effect)
Itraconazole	Oral solution associated with gastrointestinal adverse effects, including nausea, vomiting, and osmotic diarrhea due to cyclodextrin component; increases in liver function tests reported and possibility of hepatotoxiciy; negative inotropic effects have been reported (avoid use in evidence of ventricular dysfunction such as congestive heart failure)
Posaconazole	Generally well-tolerated; increases in liver function tests and possibility of hepatotoxicity; QTc prolongation has been observed on electrocardiogram
Voriconazole	Transient visual disturbances (hallucinations, photophobia, color changes, halo effect) associated with intravenous administration; optic neuritis and papilledema may occur with prolonged therapy (>28 days); photosensitivity and skin reactions, including rashes and exfoliative cutaneous reactions may occur; encephalopathy reported with elevated trough levels (>5.5 μg/mL); increases in liver function tests reported and possibility of hepatotoxicity; QTc prolongation has also been observed on electrocardiogram; intravenous formulation formulated with cyclodextrin (caution in patients with renal impairment)
Echinocandins	
Anidulafungin	Generally well-tolerated; infusion-related reactions associated with histamine release may occur with initial dose
Caspofungin	Generally well-tolerated; infusion-related reactions associated with histamine release may occur with initial dose; asymptomatic increases in liver function tests may occur (usually ≤3× ULN)
Micafungin	Generally well-tolerated; infusion-related reactions associated with histamine release may occur with initial dose; asymptomatic increases in liver function tests may occur (usually ≤3× ULN)
Amphotericin B Formulations	
Amphotericin B deoxycholate	Significant infusion-related reactions can occur beginning with first dose, including fever, chills, arthralgias, myalgias, and rigors. Bronchospasm, hypotension, arrhythmias, apnea, and anaphylaxis less common; nephrotoxicity is most significant delayed and dose-limiting toxicity (hypokalemia, hypomagnesemia, azotemia, renal tubular acidosis; renal failure may occur)
Amphotericin B colloidal dispersion	Nephrotoxicity may be reduced compared with deoxycholate formulation but is not eliminated; similar rates of infusion-related reactions to amphotericin B deoxycholate; hypoxic episodes with fever and chills associated with infusion
Amphotericin B lipid complex	Infusion-related reactions and nephrotoxicity may be reduced compared with deoxycholate formulation, but are not eliminated
Liposomal amphotericin B	Infusion-related reactions and nephrotoxicity may be reduced compared with deoxycholate formulation, but are not eliminated; substernal chest discomfort and flank pain associated with therapy; sense of impending doom has also been reported with infusion
Other Agents	
Flucytosine	Neutropenia secondary to bone-marrow toxicity observed with prolonged plasma peak concentrations above 100 μg/mL; hepatotoxicity, nausea, and vomiting also can occur
Terbinafine	Increases in liver function tests and hepatotoxicity, including hepatic failure, may occur with use; taste and smell disturbances, including severe and permanent effects, have been reported

[a]Hepatotoxicity, including cases of hepatic failure, has been reported with each of the azoles; the azoles are also teratogenic and should be avoided during pregnancy.

TABLE 2.3.3 Treatment of Superficial Fungal Infections

Infection	Topical Therapy	Systemic Therapy	Comments
Candida			
Oropharyngeal candidiasis	• Clotrimazole troches 10 mg five times daily • Nystatin suspension QID	• Fluconazole 100–200 mg/day • Itraconazole solution 200 mg/day • Posaconazole 400 mg/day • Voriconazole 200 mg/day • An echinocandin • Amphotericin B deoxycholate 0.3 mg/kg/day • Amphotericin B deoxycholate oral suspension	• Fluconazole is recommended for moderate-to-severe oropharyngeal candidiasis; uncomplicated disease is treated for 7–14 days; intravenous fluconazole, an echinocandin, or amphotericin B deoxycholate can be used in patients unable to tolerate oral agents (*Clin Inf Dis.* 2009;48:503)
Vulvovaginal candidiasis	• Butoconazole cream QD x 3 days • Clotrimazole cream × 1 • Miconazole cream × 1 or 100 mg suppository × 7 days or 200 mg suppository × 3 days • Tioconazole 2% cream × 3 days or 6.5% cream × 1	• Fluconazole 150 mg × 1	
Cutaneous Mycoses			
Tinea pedis, tinea manuum, tinea cruris, and tinea corporis	• Butenafine or econazole QD • Ciclopirox, clotrimazole, haloprogin, ketoconazole, miconazole, naftifine, oxiconazole, sulconazole, terbinafine or tolnaftate BID	• Fluconazole 150 mg weekly × 4 weeks • Ketoconazole 200 mg QD × 4 weeks • Itraconazole 200–400 mg QD × 1 week • Terbinafine 250 mg QD × 2 weeks	• 2–4 weeks of therapy adequate for mild infections; severe infections may require prolonged treatment

(Continued)

TABLE 2.3.3 Treatment of Superficial Fungal Infections *(Continued)*

Infection	Topical Therapy	Systemic Therapy	Comments
Tinea capitis	Shampoo (ketoconazole, selenium sulfide, povidone-iodine) in conjunction with oral therapy	Terbinafine 250 mg QD × 4–8 weeks	• Shampoo alone may be used in asymptomatic carriers
Onychomycosis (fingernails)	Ciclopirox 8% nail lacquer, apply nightly for up to 48 weeks	• Fluconazole 50 mg QD or 300 mg once weekly for 6 (finger) or 12 (toe) months • Itraconazole 200 mg QD × 6 (finger) or 12 (toe) weeks or 200 mg BID × 1 week and repeated 4 weeks after initial treatment (finger) or repeated at 4 and 8 weeks (toe) or • Terbinafine 250 mg QD × 6 (finger) or 12 (toe) weeks	• Usually secondary to dermatophytes, may be caused by candida in immunosuppressed patients • More common in toenails than fingernails

Sources: (1) Pappas PG, Kauffman CA, Andes D, Benjamin DK, Calandra TF, (2) Edwards JE, et al. Clinical practice guidelines for the management of candidiasis: 2009 update by the Infectious Diseases Society of America. *Clin Inf Dis.* 2009;48:503–535; (3) Brown TE, Dresser LD, Chin TW. Superficial fungal infections. In: Dipiro JT, Talbert RL, Matzke GR, Posey LM, Wells BG, Yee GC, eds. *Pharmacotherapy: A Pathophysiologic Approach.* 8th ed. New York, NY: McGraw-Hill; 2011:chap. 29.

TABLE 2.3.4 Treatment of Invasive Fungal Infections

Condition	Therapy	Comments
Aspergillosis		
Invasive pulmonary aspergillosis	Primary: • Voriconazole 6 mg/kg every 12 h for 1 day, then 4 mg/kg every 12 h (oral dose 200–300 mg) Alternative: • LAMB 3–5 mg/kg/day • ABLC 5 mg/kg/day • Caspofungin 70 mg loading dose, then 50 mg/day • Posaconazole 200 mg QID, then 400 mg BID once stable	• Treatment of other aspergillosis conditions (e.g., sinus, tracheobronchial, CNS, endocarditis, endophthalmitis) similar to invasive pulmonary aspergillosis • Prolonged therapy and the use of other modalities may be required
Empiric or preemptive therapy	Primary • LAMB 3 mg/kg/day • Caspofungin 70 mg loading dose, then 50 mg/day • Itraconazole 200 mg/day IV or 200 mg BID PO • Voriconazole 6 mg/kg every 12 h for 1 day, then 4 mg/kg every 12 h (oral dose 200)	
Prophylaxis	Primary Posaconazole 200 mg every 8 h Alternative: • Itraconazole 200 mg every 12 h IV for 2 days, then 200 mg/day IV, or 200 mg PO every 12 h; • Micafungin 50 mg/day	
Blastomycosis		
Pulmonary	Mild to moderate—itraconazole 200 mg QD or BID for 6 months–1 year Moderately severe to severe—lipid amphotericin B 3–5 mg/kg/day or amphotericin B deoxycholate 0.7–1 mg/kg/day for 1–2 weeks, then itraconazole 200 mg BID for 6 months–1 year	

(Continued)

TABLE 2.3.4 Treatment of Invasive Fungal Infections (*Continued*)

Condition	Therapy	Comments
Disseminated	Mild to moderate—itraconazole 200 mg QD or BID for 6 months–1 year Moderately severe to severe—lipid amphotericin B 3–5 mg/kg/day or amphotericin B deoxycholate 0.7–1 mg/kg/day for 1–2 weeks, then itraconazole 200 mg BID for 1 year	
CNS	Lipid amphotericin B 5 mg/kg/day for 4–6 weeks, followed by an oral azole for ≥1 year (e.g., fluconazole 800 mg/day, itraconazole 200 mg BID or TID, or voriconazole 200–400 mg BID)	
Immunosuppressed patients	Lipid amphotericin B 3–5 mg/kg/day or amphotericin B deoxycholate 0.7–1 mg/kg/day for 1–2 weeks followed by itraconazole 200 mg BID for 1 year (lifelong suppressive therapy may be required if immunosuppression not reversed)	
Pregnant women	Lipid amphotericin B 3–5 mg/kg/day	
Candidiasis		
Empiric treatment of suspected candidiasis in non-neutropenic patients	Primary • Fluconazole 12 mg/kg loading dose (800 mg), then 6 mg/kg/day (400 mg) • An echinocandin Secondary • Lipid amphotericin B 3–5 mg/kg/day	• Consider empiric antifungal therapy after 4 days of persistent fever despite antibiotics in neutropenic patients • Avoid azoles in patients with prior azole prophylaxis
Empiric treatment of suspected candidiasis in neutropenic patients	Primary • Lipid amphotericin B 3–5 mg/kg/day • Caspofungin 70 mg loading dose, then 50 mg daily Secondary • Voriconazole 6 mg/kg BID × 2 (400 mg), then 3 mg/kg (200 mg) BID • Fluconazole 12 mg/kg loading dose (800 mg), then 6 mg/kg/day (400 mg)	

Candidemia (non-neutropenic patients)	**Primary** • Fluconazole 12 mg/kg loading dose (800 mg), then 6 mg/kg/day (400 mg); • An echinocandin **Secondary** • Lipid amphotericin B 3–5 mg/kg/day • Voriconazole 6 mg/kg BID × 2 (400 mg), then 3 mg/kg (200 mg) BID	• An echinocandin is preferred for moderate severe to severe illness and in patients with recent azole exposure • Fluconazole recommended for those who are not critically ill and without recent azole exposure • Treatment should continue for 14 days after first negative blood culture and resolution of signs and symptoms
Candidemia (neutropenic patients)	**Primary** • An echinocandin • Lipid amphotericin B 3–5 mg/kg/day **Alternative** • Fluconazole 12 mg/kg loading dose (800 mg), then 6 mg/kg/day (400 mg) • Voriconazole 6 mg/kg BID × 2 (400 mg), then 3 mg/kg (200 mg) BID	• Treat for candidemia in patients with pyelonephritis and suspected disseminated candidiasis
Symptomatic cystitis	**Primary** • Fluconazole 200 mg/day for 2 weeks **Alternative** • Amphotericin B deoxycholate 0.3–0.6 mg/kg/day for 1–7 days	
Pyelonephritis	**Primary** • Fluconazole 3–6 mg/kg/day (200–400 mg) for 2 weeks **Alternative** • Amphotericin B deoxycholate 0.5–0.7 mg/kg/day ± flucytosine 25 mg/kg QID for 2 weeks	

(Continued)

TABLE 2.3.4 Treatment of Invasive Fungal Infections *(Continued)*

Condition	Therapy	Comments
Esophageal candidiasis	**Primary** • Fluconazole 3–6 mg/kg/day (200–400 mg) • An echinocandin • Amphotericin B deoxycholate 0.3–0.7 mg/kg/day **Alternative** • Itraconazole oral solution 200 mg/day • Posaconazole 400 mg BID • Voriconazole 200 mg BID	• Treat for 14–21 days
Chronic disseminated candidiasis	**Primary** • Fluconazole 6 mg/kg/day (400 mg) if patient stable • Lipid amphotericin B 3–5 mg/kg/day for severely ill patients **Alternative** • An echinocandin for several weeks followed by fluconazole	• Treatment should continue through periods of immunosuppression and should continue until lesions resolve (usually months)
Candida endophthalmitis	**Primary** • Amphotericin B deoxycholate 0.7–1 mg/kg/day with flucytosine 25 mg/kg QID • Fluconazole 6–12 mg/kg/day **Alternative** • Lipid amphotericin B 3–5 mg/kg/day • Voriconazole 6 mg/kg every 12 h for 2 doses, then 4 mg/kg every 12 h	• Surgical intervention for patients with severe endophthalmitis or vitreitis • Treat for 4–6 weeks
Coccidioidomycosis		
Uncomplicated pneumonia	• No treatment or fluconazole 400 mg/day or itraconazole 200 mg BID for 3–6 months (3 months after resolution of clinical infection) • With risk of dissemination or severe disease, fluconazole ≥400 mg/day or itraconazole ≥200 mg BID for 3–6 months (≥3 months after resolution of clinical infection); follow all patients closely	

Pulmonary cavity	• Observation or fluconazole 400 mg/day for 6–12 months; • Treatment recommended in patients with chronic progressive fibrocavitary disease (therapy for at least 1 year in duration)
Progressive pulmonary of disseminated nonmeningeal	• Life threatening—amphotericin B deoxycholate 0.6–1.0 mg/kg/day or lipid amphotericin B 3–5 mg/kg/day, and transition to fluconazole or itraconazole when disease controlled (duration of therapy at least 2 years) • Slowly progressive or stable—fluconazole ≥400 mg/day or itraconazole ≥200 mg BID (duration at least 2 years)
Meningitis	• Fluconazole ≥400 mg/day (some physicians may advocate doses of ≥800 mg) or itraconazole ≥200 mg BID; • Intrathecal amphotericin B (0.1 to 1.5 mg/dose from intervals of daily to week[a]) in combination with an azole has been used (begin at low dosage) • Patients with coccidioidal meningitis may continue lifelong antifungal therapy due to high relapse rate
HIV-positive patients	• Treatment is recommended for all HIV-positive patients with CD4 count ≤250 cells/μL and continued as long as CD4 counts above this level
Pregnant patients	• Primary infection during pregnancy or immediately postpartum may prompt initiation of treatment • Amphotericin B should be used in pregnancy due to teratogenic effects of azoles
Cryptococcus	
Meningitis—induction	• Amphotericin B deoxycholate 0.7–1.0 mg/kg/day + flucytosine 25 mg/kg QID for 2 weeks (HIV patients) or 4 weeks (non-HIV, nontransplant patients) • LAMB 3–4 mg/kg/day or ABLC 5 mg/kg/day + flucytosine 25 mg/kg QID for 2 weeks (HIV, transplant patients)	• May substitute lipid formulation for amphotericin B deoxycholate for 2nd 2 weeks of induction in non-HIV, nontransplant patients • Flucytosine-free induction regimens: extend amphotericin B deoxycholate to 6 weeks (nontransplant); ABLC or LAMB therapy to 6 weeks (HIV) or increase LAMB dose to 6 mg/kg/day for 6 weeks (transplant)
Meningitis—consolidation	• Fluconazole 400 mg/day for 8 weeks (HIV patients) • Fluconazole 400–800 mg/day for 8 weeks (transplant, non-HIV patients)	

(Continued)

TABLE 2.3.4 Treatment of Invasive Fungal Infections *(Continued)*

Condition	Therapy	Comments
Meningitis—maintenance	• Fluconazole 200 mg/day for ≥1 year (HIV patients) or 6 months–1 year (non-HIV, non-transplant patients) • Fluconazole 200–400 mg/day for 6 months–1 year (transplant patients)	
Pulmonary, mild-to-moderate	• Fluconazole 400 mg/day for 6 months–1 year	
Pulmonary, severe or cryptococcemia	• Treat as meningitis	
Histoplasmosis		
Acute pulmonary	• Mild to moderate and symptoms >4 weeks—itraconazole 200 mg TID for 3 days, then 200 mg QD or BID for 6–12 weeks • Moderately severe or severe—lipid amphotericin B 3–5 mg/kg/day or amphotericin B deoxycholate 0.7–1.0 mg/kg/day for 2 weeks, then itraconazole 200 mg/day for 12 additional weeks	• Chronic suppressive therapy required in HIV/AIDS patients who do not achieve immune reconstitution with antiretroviral therapy; this may also be needed in other patients with immunosuppressive disorders and in those who relapse despite appropriate therapy • Monitoring of itraconazole serum levels should be considered in patients being treated for chronic pulmonary, disseminated, or CNS histoplasmosis; a random serum concentration of >1.0 µg/mL should be achieved
Chronic cavitary pulmonary	• Itraconazole 200 mg TID for 3 days, then 200 mg BID for ≥1 year • Amphotericin B deoxycholate 0.7 mg/kg/day for 12–16 weeks	
Progress disseminated	• Moderately severe to severe—lipid amphotericin B 3–5 mg/kg/day for 2 weeks, then 200 mg TID for 3 days, then 200 mg BID for ≥1 year • Mild to moderate—itraconazole 200 mg TID for 3 days, then 200 mg BID for ≥1 year	
CNS	• Lipid amphotericin B 5 mg/kg/day for a 4–6 weeks (up to a total of 175 mg/kg), then itraconazole 200 mg BID or TID daily for ≥1 year	

TABLE 2.3.5 Antifungal Drug Interactions

Antifungal	Interacting Drugs	Comments
Azoles[a]		
Fluconazole	Warfarin, rifampin	CYP isoenzyme inhibition by fluconazole increases with higher doses; rifampin significantly reduces fluconazole concentrations
Itraconazole	Midazolam, nisoldipine, pimozide, quinidine, dofetilide, triazolam, lovastatin, simvastatin, ergot alkaloids, warfarin, rifampin proton pump inhibitors H2 blockers	Inhibitors inducers of CYP 3A4 affect metabolism of itraconazole; co-administration with drugs that prolong the QT interval may result in Torsades de pointes; rhabdomyolysis may occur with HMG CoA-reductase inhibitors; co-administration may result in toxic concentrations of the calcineurin inhibitors cyclosporine tacrolimus; co-administration of proton pump inhibitors H2 blockers may significant reduce the oral bioavailability of itraconazole
Posaconazole	Sirolimus, pimozide, quinidine, lovastatin, simvastatin, ergot alkaloids, cyclosporine, tacrolimus, midazolam, warfarin, rifampin/ rifabutin, efavirenz, proton pump inhibitors, and H2 blockers	Drugs that induce UDP-glucuronidase phenytoin, rifampin/rifabutin, efavirenz) will significantly reduce posaconazole concentrations; co-administration with drugs that prolong the QTc interval may result in Torsades de pointes; rhabdomyolysis may occur with HMG CoA-reductase inhibitors; co-administration may result in toxic concentrations of the calcineurin inhibitors cyclosporine and tacrolimus; co-administration of proton pump inhibitors and H2 blockers may significantly reduce the oral bioavailability of posaconazole
Voriconazole	Rifampin/rifabutin, carbamazepine, long acting barbiturates, St. John's wort, sirolimus, ergot alkaloids, cyclosporine, tacrolimus, warfarin	Inhibitors and inducers of CYP 2C9, 2C- 9, and 3A4 affect metabolism of voriconazole; co-administration with drugs that prolong the QTc interval may result in Torsades de pointes; rhabdomyolysis may occur with HMG CoA-reductase inhibitors; co-administration may result in toxic concentrations of the calcineurin inhibitors cyclosporine and tacrolimus

(Continued)

TABLE 2.3.5 Antifungal Drug Interactions (*Continued*)

Antifungal	Interacting Drugs	Comments
Echinocandins		
Anidulafungin	Cyclosporine	The echinocandins are not clinically relevant substrates, inducers, or inhibitors of CYP450 isoenzymes; cyclosporine may cause increases in echinocandin exposures (i.e., AUC); inducers of drug clearance (e.g., rifampin and phenytoin) may increase bloodstream clearance of caspofungin (consider increasing daily dose to 70 mg); caspofungin may reduce tacrolimus concentrations (monitor tacrolimus levels); sirolimus and nifedipine concentrations (C_{max} and AUC) may be increased by micafungin
Caspofungin	Cyclosporine, tacrolimus, rifampin, nevirapine, efavirenz, phenytoin, dexamethasone, carbamazepine	
Micafungin	Sirolimus, nifedipine	
Polyenes		
Amphotericin B formulations	Nephrotoxic agents, flucytosine, digoxin	Amphotericin B may potentiate the adverse renal effects of other nephrotoxic agents; amphotericin B may also reduce the clearance of renally eliminated agents (e.g., flucytosine) resulting in toxic concentrations of these agents; hypokalemia caused by amphotericin B may potentiate the toxicity of digoxin
Miscellaneous		
Flucytosine	Nephrotoxic agents	Nephrotoxic drugs may reduce the clearance of flucytosine resulting in toxic concentrations and adverse effects
Terbinafine	Tricyclic antidepressants, SSRIs, beta blockers, rifampin/rifabutin	Inhibitors and inducers of CYP2C9 and 3A4 affect the metabolism of terbinafine

[a]The azoles are potent inhibitors of CYP450 isoenzymes; co-administration of drugs that prolong the QTc interval and are metabolized via CYP450 isoenzymes are contraindicated with the azoles.

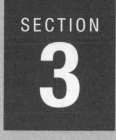

SECTION 3

Endocrinology

ABBREVIATIONS

DKA	Diabetic ketoacidosis	GLP-1	Glucagon-like peptide-1
DM	Diabetes mellitus	HbA_{1c}	Hemoglobin A_{1c}
DPP-4	Dipeptidyl peptidase-4	MNT	Medical nutrition therapy
DSC	Digoxin serum concentration	TPOab	Thyroperoxidase antibodies
FT4	Free T4	TSH	Thyroid-stimulating hormone
GIP	Gastric inhibitory peptide		

FIGURE 3.1.1 Pharmacotherapy for Diabetes

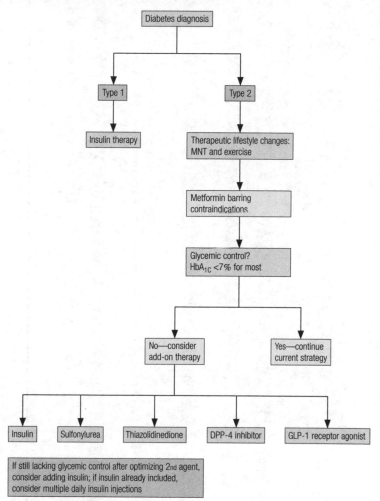

Source: Inzucchi SE, Bergenstal RM, Buse JB, et al. Management of hyperglycemia in type 2 diabetes: A patient centered approach. Position statement of the American Diabetes Association (ADA) and the European Association for the Study of Diabetes (EASD). *Diabetes Care*. 2012;35:1364.

TABLE 3.1.2 Insulins

Insulin	Onset	Peak	Duration	Considerations
Rapid Acting				
Aspart (NovoLog)	0.25–0.5 h	0.5–1.5 h	<5 h	• Inject immediately prior to meal (some patients dose with or after meal)
Glulisine (Apidra)				• Do not use IV: increased cost with no advantage vs. regular
Lispro (Humalog)		0.5–2 h		
Short Acting				
Regular	0.5–1 h	2–4 h	5–8 h	• Inject ~30 min prior to eating
Intermediate				
NPH (Humulin N, Novolin N)	1–2 h	4–10 h	10–18 h	• Peak and duration highly variable, especially in elderly; be aware of nocturnal hypoglycemia
Long Acting				
Glargine (Lantus)	1.5–4 h	No peak	24 h	• Some patients do not get full 24 h effect and require BID dosing • Burning at injection site—pH 4.0
Detemir (Levemir)		Slow steady rise ~3–4 h	<0.4 units/kg highly variable; <24 h; >0.4 units/kg ~24 h	• Administer BID for low doses (<0.4 units/kg) • Only insulin to show (minor) weight loss vs. gain (*Diabetes Care.* 2011;34:1487)
Combination Products				
70% aspart protamine/30% aspart	0.25–0.5 h	Dual peak	10–16 h	• Longer-acting insulin always listed 1st • Time to onset determined by faster-acting insulin; duration by intermediate insulin
50% lispro protamine/50% lispro				
75% lispro protamine/25% lispro				
70% NPH/30% regular	0.5–1 h		10–18 h	

TABLE 3.1.3 Selected Non-Insulin Antihyperglycemic Agents

Class	Drug (Brand)	Dosing	Comments
α-Glucosidase inhibitors	Acarbose[a] (Precose) 25, 50, 100 mg tabs Miglitol (Glyset) 25, 50, 100 mg tabs	25 mg QD–TID @ meals w/1st bite of food, titrate Q 4–8 weeks; adjust based on 1° postprandial glucose; 100 mg TID max	• MOA: Enzyme inhibitor, delays hydrolysis of complex carbohydrates • 0.5–0.8% decrease in A_{1c} • Contraindications: Renal dysfunction (Scr ≥ 2 mg/dL); inflammatory bowel disease; GI obstruction • AEs: Flatulence, diarrhea, abdominal pain, may avoid through slow titration; acarbose ~14% have ↑ AST/ALT – monitor Q 3 months • Dosing requirements may decrease compliance
Biguanide	Metformin[a] (glucophage, glucophage XL) 500, 850, 1,000 mg tabs; 500, 750, 1,000 mg XR tabs	IR 500 mg BID; increase by 500 mg Q week up to 2550 mg/day (850 mg TID) XR 500–1,000 mg/day max 2,500 mg/day; if not controlled with max dose, split BID	• Decrease hepatic glucose production and intestinal glucose absorption; increases insulin sensitivity • 1–2% decrease in A_{1c} • Contraindicated in renal dysfunction (Scr ≥1.5 mg/dL males, ≥1.4 mg/dL females); acute/chronic acidosis; discontinue in AKI or if patient to receive contrast • Considered weight neutral—typically causes weight loss • AEs: Abdominal pain, cramping, flatulence; GI effects worse with IR vs. XR; take w/food and titrate slowly, B_{12} deficiency
Bile acid sequestrant	Colesevelam (Welchol) 3.75 g/packet granules for suspension, 625 mg tabs	Combination therapy: 3.75 g QD, 1.875 g BID	• MOA: Unknown, may decrease glucose absorption and hepatic glucose production and increase GLP-1 • 0.5–0.7% decrease in A_{1c} • AEs: Constipation • Separate from other meds—binding may decrease absorption • Large tablet size/pill burden • LDL decrease 15–19%; increases triglycerides

(Continued)

TABLE 3.1.3 Selected Non-Insulin Antihyperglycemic Agents (Continued)

Class	Drug (Brand)	Dosing	Comments
D₂ agonist	Bromocriptine (Cycloset) 0.8 mg tabs	0.8 mg QAM; titrate by 0.8 mg Q week up to 4.8 mg/day	• MOA: Unknown, believed to reset circadian rhythm and reverse insulin resistance • 0.6–0.9% decrease in A₁c • Contraindicated with α, β agonists, azole antifungals; risk of serotonin syndrome with serotonergic agents; caution with psychiatric history • Extensive hepatic metabolism • AEs: Increased CNS effects including dizziness, HA, fatigue, drowsiness; hypotension, syncope; GI upset—take with food
DPP-IV inhibitors	Linagliptin (Tradjenta) 5 mg tabs	5 mg QD; no renal adjustments	• MOA: Inhibits enzyme responsible for metabolism of incretin hormones and increased [GLP-1], [GIP] • 0.5–0.8% decrease in A₁c
	Saxagliptin (Onglyza) 2.5, 5 mg tabs	2.5–5 mg QD; CrCl <50 mL/min: 2.5 mg QD	• AEs: Headache, peripheral edema, hemorrhagic pancreatitis • Weight neutral
	Sitagliptin (Januvia) 25, 50, 100 mg tabs	100 mg QD; CrCl ≥30–50 mL/min: 50 mg QD; CrCl <30 mL/min: 25 mg QD	• Linagliptin, saxagliptin—CYP3A4 substrates; decrease saxagliptin to 2.5 mg QD w/strong 3A4 inhibitor
GLP-1 agonists	Liraglutide (Victoza) 6 mg/ mL soln; 3 mL pen	0.6 mg SQ QD × 1 week, then 1.2 mg SQ QD; may titrate to 1.8 mg QD	• MOA: GLP-1 analog, increases glucose-dependent insulin secretion, decreases glucagon secretion, delays gastric emptying and increases satiety
	Exenatide (Byetta) 250 µg/ mL soln; 2.4 mL = 60 IR doses; (Bydureon) 2 mg soln = 1 XR dose	IR–5 µg within 60 min of meal; 10 µg BID after 1 month if needed; XR–2 mg Q week CrCl <30 mL/min not recommended	• 0.5–1.0% decrease in A₁c; 1.5–1.9% decrease in A₁c–XR exenatide • Weight loss • Contraindications: Multiple endocrine neoplasia syndrome type 2; family history of medullary thyroid carcinoma • AEs: N/V/D, dose-related, decreases with exposure, hemorrhagic pancreatitis, injection side irritation

Meglitinides	Nateglinide[a] (Starlix) 60, 120 mg tabs	120 mg TID	• MOA: Stimulates glucose-dependent insulin release • 0.5–1.5% decrease in A_{1c} • Weight gain (↑insulin secretion) • Take within 15–30 min of meal; skip dose if skip meal • AEs: Hypoglycemia
	Repaglinide (Prandin) 0.5, 1, 2 mg tabs	Initial: 0.5 mg (untreated or A_{1c} <8%); 1–2 mg (prior treatment or A_{1c}>8%); max 4 mg/dose (16 mg/day) CrCl 20–40 mL/min: initiate @ 0.5 mg/dose	• Nateglinide—CYP 2C9/3A4 substrate; CI—conivaptan • Repaglinide—CYP3A4/2C8 substrate; CI—conivaptan; also metabolized via glucuronidation; CI—gemfibrozil
Sulfonylureas	Glimepiride[a] (Amaryl) 1, 2, 4 mg tabs	1–2 mg QAM with breakfast (or 1st meal); max 8 mg/day	• MOA: Stimulates pancreatic insulin release, decreases hepatic glucose production • 1–2% decrease in A_{1c}
	Glipizide[a] (Glucotrol) 5, 10 mg tabs	IR–5 mg QD; 40 mg max; divide doses >15 mg	• Weight gain (↑insulin secretion) • AE: Dizziness, HA, hypoglycemia (>w/↑age)
	(Glucotrol XL) 2.5, 5, 10 mg XR tabs	XR–5 mg QD; 20 mg max CrCl <50 mL/min: decrease dose by 50%	• Sulfonylureas associated w/ increased CV mortality vs. diet/insulin • Caution in sulfonamide allergy, G6PD deficiency
	Glyburide[a] (DiaBeta) 1.25, 2.5, 5 mg tabs (Micronase) 1.5, 3, 6 mg micronized tabs	Regular tabs ≠ micronized tabs 2.5–5 mg (1.5–3 mg micronized) initial; max 20 mg/day (12 mg/day micronized); max doses more effective if divided; CrCl <50 mL/min not recc	• Glimepiride, glipizide—CYP2C9 substrates, metabolites excreted in urine • Secondary failure common with beta-cell destruction; pancreas unable to continue insulin production
Thiazolidinediones	Pioglitazone (Actos) 15, 30, 45 mg tabs	15–30 mg QD; max 45 mg	• MOA: PPAR-gamma agonists; increases insulin sensitivity • 0.5–1.4% decrease in A_{1c} • Weight gain
	Rosiglitazone (Avandia) 2, 4, 8 mg tabs	4 mg QD; max 8 mg/day (better results if divided)	• AEs: Edema (up to 15%), HF, HA, increases fracture risk (rosi >> pio) • Pioglitazone: Increased risk of bladder cancer • Rosiglitazone: Increased risk of MI • Increased HDL (rosi and pio); Increased LDL (rosi)

(Continued)

TABLE 3.1.3 Selected Non-Insulin Antihyperglycemic Agents *(Continued)*

Class	Drug (Brand)	Dosing	Comments
Amylinomimetic	Pramlintide (Symlin, SymlinPen 60, SymlinPen 120) 1,000 µg/mL; 1.5 mL (60 pen), 2.7 mL (120 pen) injectors	DM1–15 µg SQ just prior to meals; titrate Q 3 days (if nausea tolerable) target 30–60 µg DM2–15 µg SQ just prior to meals; titrate Q 3 days (if nausea tolerable) target 30–60 µg	• MOA: Amylin analog; delays gastric emptying, centrally mediated appetite suppression, decreases glucagon secretion • 0.5–1.0% decrease in A$_{1c}$ • Weight loss (secondary to decreased intake) • Decrease insulin 50% at initiation to mitigate risk of hypoglycemia • AEs: Severe hypoglycemia, N/V, gastroparesis, HA, • Contraindications: Gastroparesis, hypoglycemic unawareness (caution w/ beta blockers secondary to masking hypoglycemic symptoms)

AEs—hypoglycemia listed only for products that frequently cause hypoglycemia as monotherapy.

Source: Inzucchi SE, Bergenstal RM, Buse JB, et al. Management of hyperglycemia in type 2 diabetes: A patient centered approach. Position statement of the American Diabetes Association (ADA) and the European Association for the Study of Diabetes (EASD). *Diabetes Care.* 2012;35:1364.

^{a}Generic available.

TABLE 3.1.4 Hyperglycemic Crises

Criteria	DKA	HHS

Pathophysiology	• Insulin deficiency leads to lipolysis (breakdown of adipose tissue to free fatty acids) for energy production, ketone formation, and metabolic acidosis
	• Precipitating factors—develops quickly
	  • Illness/Infection
	  • Inadequate insulin
	  • Initial presentation of diabetes (type 1 typically)
		• Residual insulin protects against lipolysis; peripheral muscle tissue used for energy production, no ketones
		• Precipitating factors—develops slowly
		  • Undiagnosed/untreated DM
		  • Illness/Infection

Presentation	• Signs/symptoms
	  • N/V, abdominal cramps
	  • Polyuria, polydipsia, polyphagia
	  • Kussmaul's respirations
	  • Mental status changes
	  • Fruity "ketone breath"
		• Signs/symptoms
		  • Similar to DKA; milder GI symptoms
		  • No Kussmaul's respirations
		  • Mental status changes common
		  • Typically profound dehydration

Glucose	>250 mg/dL	>600 mg/dL
pH (arterial)	<7.2	>7.3
Serum bicarbonate	<15 mEq/L	>18 mEq/L
Serum/urine ketones	+	−/Small
Anion gap	↑	Variable
Potassium	Variable; total body depletion	Variable; total body depletion
Water deficit	5–7 L	7–12 L

(Continued)

TABLE 3.1.4 Hyperglycemic Crises *(Continued)*

Treatment

Volume

- Expand extracellular volume/restore renal perfusion
  - 15–20 mL/kg NS, ½ NS
  - Switch to D_5W + ½ NS when glucose ≈ 200–250 mg/dL

Electrolytes

- Assess hydration state, electrolyte levels and urinary output
  - K^+ <5.3 mEq/L
  - Initiate after urinary output verified; before/with insulin in DKA → insulin will worsen existing hypokalemia by shifting K^+ intracellularly
  - Bicarbonate replacement controversial, may be detrimental
  - Consider if pH <7.0

Glycemic control

- Use regular insulin *only*; rapid acting insulins do NOT offer any benefit; increased cost
  - Optional bolus: 0.1 units/kg
  - Infusion 0.1 units/kg/h (5–10 units/h)
  - Slow steady fall in glucose ~50–75 mg/dL/h
  - Goal 200–250 mg/dL—do NOT stop insulin at this point
  - Initiate D_5W + ½ NS and continue insulin infusion to allow ketones to clear (close anion gap)

FIGURE 3.2.1 Hyperthyroidism Pharmacotherapy Algorithm

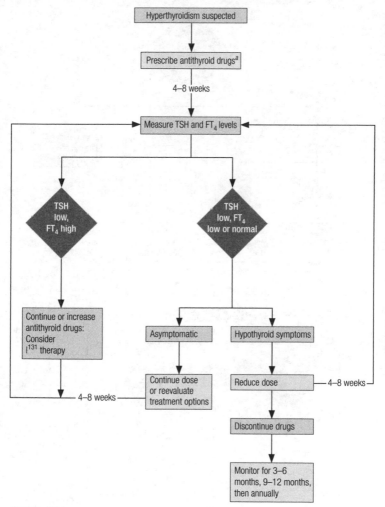

ᵃSee table 3.2.4

FIGURE 3.2.2 Hypothyroidism Pharmacotherapy Algorithm

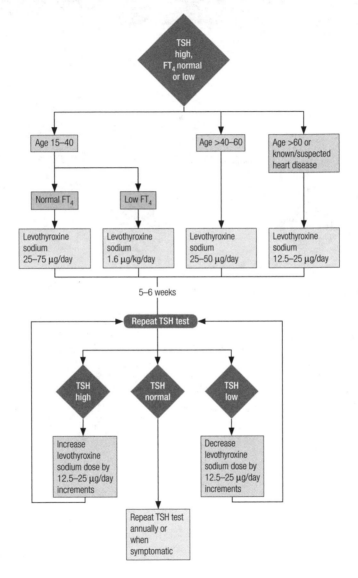

TABLE 3.2.3 Thyroid Replacement Products

Product	Source	Relative Potency	Comments
Desiccated thyroid USP (Armour Thyroid, and others)	Desiccated pork or beef thyroid	1 grain (65 mg)	• Hormone content variable; generic brands may not be bioequivalent
Levothyroxine (Levoxyl, Synthroid, Unithroid, and others)	Synthetic T_4	60 µg PO 30 µg IV	• Predictable potency; when switching from natural thyroid to L-thyroxine, lower dose by 1/2 grain; variable absorption between products; half-life = 7 days, so daily dosing; considered to be drug of choice
Liothyronine (Cytomel)	Synthetic T_3	15 µg PO and IV	• Rarely needed, rapid onset, no outcome benefit vs. T_4
Liotrix (Thyrolar)	Synthetic T_4 and T_3 in 4:1 ratio	50 µg T_4 and 12.5 µg T_3	• Potential for toxicity from high T_3 content

TABLE 3.2.4 Drugs for Hyperthyroidism

Drug	Dosing	Comments
Thionamides		
Methimazole (Tapazole)	Initial: 15–30 mg QD Maintenance: 5–10 mg QD Thyroid storm: 60–120 mg QD	• Thionamides 1st line drugs for Grave's disease • Warfarin and clotting factor metabolism decreases as patient becomes euthyroid, monitor INR closely • Digoxin metabolism decreases as patient becomes euthyroid, monitor DSC
Propylthiouracil (PTU)	Initial: 300 mg TID Maintenance: 100–200 mg QD Thyroid storm: 600–1200 mg QD	• Methimazole induces more rapid decrease in T3 and T4 levels than PTU (*J Clin Endocrinol Metab* 1987;65:719.) • PTU preferred agent in first trimester pregnancy
Other Agents		
Beta-blockers	See Table 1.1.1	• Decreases symptoms from increased adrenergic tone
Cholestyramine	4 grams QID	• Decreases T3 and T4 levels in combination with methimazole faster than methimazole alone (*J Clin Endocrinol Metab* 1996;81:3191.)
Potassium iodide (SSKI)	10 drops QD	• Useful for symptom control in mild hyperthyroidism

TABLE 4.1.1 Criteria for t-PA Use in Acute Ischemic Stroke

Inclusion Criteria

All of the items below must be true in order to use t-PA:
- Age 18 years or older
- Clinical diagnosis of ischemic stroke causing a measurable neurologic deficit
- Time of symptom onset well established to be less than 4.5 hours before treatment would begin

Exclusion Criteria

All of the items below must be false in order to use t-PA:
- Evidence of intracranial hemorrhage on noncontrast head CT
- Only minor or rapidly improving stroke symptoms
- High clinical suspicion of subarachnoid hemorrhage even with normal CT
- Active internal bleeding (e.g., GI/GU bleeding within 21 days)
- Known bleeding diathesis, including but not limited to platelet count <100,000/mm^3
- Patient has received heparin within 48 hours and had an elevated APTT
- Recent use of anticoagulant (e.g., warfarin) and elevated PT (>15 second)/INR
- Intracranial surgery, serious head trauma, or previous stroke within 3 months
- Major surgery or serious trauma within 14 days
- Recent arterial puncture at noncompressible site
- Lumbar puncture within 7 days
- History of intracranial hemorrhage, arteriovenous malformation, or aneurysm
- Witnessed seizure at stroke onset
- Recent acute myocardial infarction
- SBP >185 mm Hg or DBP >110 mm Hg at time of treatment

Additional exclusion criteria if within 3–4.5 hours of onset:
- Age greater than 80 years
- Current treatment with oral anticoagulants
- NIH Stroke Scale Score >25 (severe stroke)
- History of both stroke and diabetes

Reproduced with permission from Fagan S, Hess DC. Stroke. In: Dipro JT, Talbert RL, Yee GC, Matzke GR, Wells BG, Posey LM, eds. *Pharmacotherapy. A Pathophysiologic Approach.* 8th ed. New York, NY: McGraw-Hill Companies; 2011.

FIGURE 4.1.2 Pharmacotherapy of Acute Ischemic Stroke[a]

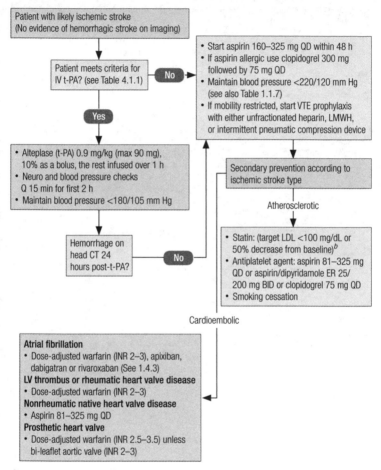

Sources: (1) Furie KL, Kasner SE, Adams RJ, et al.; on behalf of the American Heart Association Stroke Council, Council on Cardiovascular Nursing, Council on Clinical Cardiology, and Interdisciplinary Council on Quality of Care and Outcomes Research. Guidelines for the prevention of stroke in patients with stroke or transient ischemic attack: a guideline for healthcare professionals from the American Heart Association/ American Stroke Association. *Stroke.* 2011;42:227–276. (2) Lansberg MG, O'Donnell MJ, Khatri P, et al. Antithrombotic and Thrombolytic Therapy for Ischemic Stroke: Antithrombotic Therapy and Prevention of Thrombosis, 9th ed.: *American College of Chest Physicians Evidence-Based Clinical Practice Guidelines. Chest.* 2012;141:e601S–636S.
[a]See also Table 4.1.3 for details on selection and dosing of specific agents.
[b]See tables 1.3.1 and 1.3.4

TABLE 4.1.3 Pharmacotherapy for Secondary Prevention of Ischemic Stroke

Drug	Dosing	Comments
Antiplatelet Agents		
Aspirin	160–325 mg QD acutely, 81–325 mg QD thereafter	• For secondary prevention of stroke of atherosclerotic origin, AHA/ASA guidelines recommend aspirin or aspirin/dipyridamole ER as first line and clopidogrel for aspirin intolerance (*Stroke*. 2011;42:227); ACCP guidelines recommend either aspirin/dipyridamole ER or clopidogrel over aspirin due to modestly better efficacy despite higher cost (*Chest* 2012;141:e601S)
Aspirin/dipyridamole ER (Aggrenox) 25/200 mg	1 tablet BID	• Both guidelines recommend aspirin for cardioembolic source due to PFO or nonrheumatic native valve disease
Clopidogrel (Plavix) 75 mg tablet	1 tablet QD	• Aspirin plus clopidogrel may be considered for patients with atrial fibrillation who cannot take anticoagulation for reasons other than bleeding risk (*Chest*. 2012;141:e601S) but should be otherwise avoided due to a lack of efficacy and higher bleeding risk (*Lancet*. 2004;364:331)
Anticoagulants		
Warfarin	Dose to target INR	• ACCP guidelines recommend dabigatran over warfarin for secondary prevention of stroke in patients with atrial fibrillation (*Chest*. 2012;141:e601S)
Dabigatran (Pradaxa) 150 mg tablets	See table 1.4.3	• Initiate within 1–2 weeks of stroke, unless high bleeding risk; aspirin should be used until anticoagulator started unless contraindicated
Rivaroxaban (Xarelto) 15 and 20 mg tablets		
Apixiban (Eliqius) 2.5 and 5 mg tablets		
Statins		
Atorvastatin (Lipitor) 10, 20, 40 or 80 mg tablets	Choose dose to reduce LDL <100 mg/dL or by 50% (see table 1.3.1 for dosing)	• Evidence for statins supported by 1 trial of high-dose atorvastatin (*Stroke*. 2007;38:3198); thus, AHA/ASA recommends aggressive dosing (*Stroke*. 2011;42:227) • Could be a class effect at similar doses and LDL target (see table 1.3.1 for other statins)

FIGURE 4.2.1 Diagnostic Criteria for Epilepsy

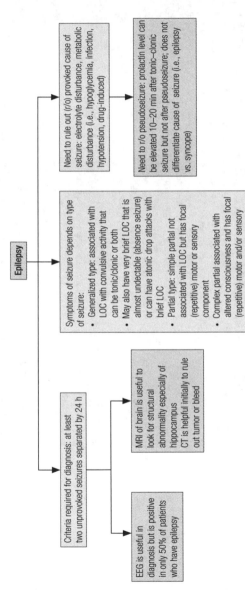

Epilepsy

Criteria required for diagnosis: at least two unprovoked seizures separated by 24 h

EEG is useful in diagnosis but is positive in only 50% of patients who have epilepsy

MRI of brain is useful to look for structural abnormality especially of hippocampus
CT is helpful initially to rule out tumor or bleed

Symptoms of seizure depends on type of seizure:
- Generalized type: associated with LOC with convulsive activity that can be tonic/clonic or both
- May also have very brief LOC that is almost undetectable (absence seizure) or can have atonic drop attacks with brief LOC
- Partial type: simple partial not associated with LOC but has focal (repetitive) motor or sensory component
- Complex partial associated with altered consciousness and has focal (repetitive) motor and/or sensory component

Need to rule out (r/o) provoked cause of seizure: electrolyte disturbance, metabolic disturbance (i.e., hypoglycemia, infection, hypotension, drug-induced)

Need to r/o pseudoseizure: prolactin level can be elevated 10–20 min after tonic–clonic seizure but not after pseudoseizure; does not differentiate cause of seizure (i.e., epilepsy vs. syncope)

FIGURE 4.2.2 Pharmacotherapy of Epilepsy

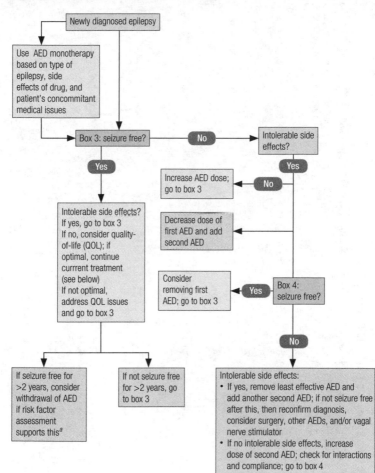

Reproduced with permission from Rogers SJ, Cavazos JE. Epilepsy. In: Dipiro JT, Talbert RL, Yee GC, Matzke GR, Wells BG, Posey LM, eds. *Pharmacotherapy. A Pathophysiologic Approach.* 8th ed. New York, NY: McGraw-Hill Companies; 2011.

[a]Favorable factors include single type of partial or primary GTC seizures, normal neurologic exam, normal IQ and an EEG that has normalized with treatment; repeated episodes of status epilepticus or history of high frequency of seizures are poor risk factors for successful withdrawal of AED.

TABLE 4.2.3 Antiepileptic Drug Dosing and Treatment Considerations

Drug		Initial Dose (Frequency), Titration, and Usual Maximum	Seizure Type	Comments
Carba	Initial	400 mg/day (BID)	Partial, primary GTC	CNS side effects including diplopia, nausea, hyponatremia, rash, blood dyscrasias
	Titration	200 mg every week		
	Maximum	400–2,400 mg/day (BID)		
Ethosuximide	Initial	500 mg/day (given BID due to GI effects)	Generalized seizures absence	CNS side effects, behavior changes, headache, blood dyscrasias
	Titration	Increase by 250 mg every 4–7 days		
	Maximum	500–2,000 mg/day (BID, higher doses TID)		
Felbamate (FBM)	Initial	1,200 mg/day (BID or TID)	Partial (refractory only), atonic seizure in Lennox–Gastaut syndrome	Anorexia, insomnia, headache, nausea, vomiting, aplastic anemia, acute hepatic failure
	Titration	Increase by 600 mg every 2 weeks		
	Maximum	3,600 mg/day (TID or QID)		
Gabapentin	Initial	900 mg/day (TID) (doses >600 mg have decreased absorption)	Partial	CNS side effects, pedal edema, weight gain
	Titration	As tolerated		
	Maximum	4,800 mg/day (QID)		
Lacosamide (Vimpat)	Initial	100 mg/day (BID)	Partial	Ataxia, dizziness, headache, nausea, vomiting, liver enzyme elevation, PR interval increase on ECG
	Titration	Increase by 100 mg every week		
	Maximum	400 mg/day (BID)		
Lamotrigine (Lamictal)	Initial	25 mg every other day if on VPA; 25–50 mg/day if not on VPA; 25–50 mg dose for patients on AED enzyme inducers) (BID, QD if XR used)	Partial, primary GTC, generalized seizure absence, JME, Lennox–Gastaut syndrome	Diplopia, dizziness, unsteadiness, rash, headache
	Titration	25 mg every week or 2 weeks (use slower titration in patient on VPA)		
	Maximum	100–500 mg if on VPA or 300–500 mg if not on VPA (BID, QD if XR used)		

Drug		Dosing	Indication	Side Effects
Levetiracetam (Keppra)	Initial	500–1,000 mg/day (BID, QD if XR used)	Partial, primary GTC, JME	Sedation, behavioral disturbance, psychosis
	Titration	Increase by 1,000 mg every 2 weeks		
	Maximum	3,000–4,000 mg/day (BID, QD if XR used)		
Oxcarbazepine (Trileptal)	Initial	300–600 mg/day (BID)	Partial, primary GTC	CNS side effects, nausea, rash, hyponatremia
	Titration	600 mg or less every week		
	Maximum	2,400–3,000 mg/day (BID)		
Phenobarbital (PB)	Initial	10–20 mg/kg loading dose, then 1–3 mg/kg/day (QD)	Partial, primary GTC	Very strong hepatic inducer, abrupt discontinuation especially dangerous, CNS side effects[a], behavior changes, cognitive impairment, metabolic bone disease, blood dyscrasias
	Titration	As tolerated		
	Maximum	180–300 mg/day (QD or BID depending on dose/tolerability)		
Phenytoin (PHT)	Initial	15–20 mg/kg load, then 3–5 mg/kg (200–400 mg) PO QD or BID or TID based on tolerability	Partial, primary GTC	CNS side effects, cognitive impairment, immunologic reactions, gingival hyperplasia, connective tissue changes blood dyscrasias, rash, cerebellar syndrome
	Titration	Increase every 7–10 days		
	Maximum	500–600 mg/day (QD or BID or TID based on tolerability and control of seizures)		
Pregabalin (Lyrica)	Initial	150 mg/day (BID or TID)	Partial	Dizziness, somnolence, blurred vision, pedal edema, behavior changes, weight gain
	Titration	As tolerated		
	Maximum	600 mg/day (BID or TID)		
Primidone	Initial	100–125 mg/day (QD)	Partial, primary GTC	Same as above especially when patient on inducer due to greater conversion to PB, not as strong hepatic inducer, first dose effect start slowly, CNS side effects, blood dyscrasias
	Titration	Increase every 3 days by 125–250 mg/d (BID or TID)		
	Maximum	750–2,000 mg/day (BID or TID)		
Rufinamide (Banzel)	Initial	400–800 mg/day (BID)	Lennox–Gastaut syndrome	Dizziness, nausea, vomiting, somnolence, multiorgan hypersensitivity, status epilepticus, leukopenia, QT shortening
	Titration	Increase by 400–800 mg every 2 days		
	Maximum	3,200 mg/day (BID)		

(Continued)

TABLE 4.2.3 Antiepileptic Drug Dosing and Treatment Considerations (Continued)

Drug	Initial Dose (Frequency), Titration, and Usual Maximum		Seizure Type	Comments
Tiagabine (Gabitril)	Initial	4–8 mg/day (QD or BID with higher dose)	Partial	CNS side effects, depression, spike-wave stupor, tremor, nervousness, weakness
	Titration	Increase by 4–8 mg every week		
	Maximum	80 mg/day (TID)		
Topiramate (Topamax)	Initial	25–50 mg/day (QD or BID if higher dose given)	Partial, primary GTC, JME, Lennox–Gastaut syndrome	Psychomotor slowing, speech or language problems, difficulty concentrating, somnolence, fatigue, dizziness, headache, metabolic acidosis, acute angle glaucoma, oligohydrosis, kidney stones, weight loss
	Titration	Increase by 25 mg every week or 2 weeks		
	Maximum	200–1,000 mg/day (BID)		
Valproic Acid (VPA)	Initial	15 mg/kg (500–1,000 mg/day) BID or TID, QD if depakote ER, BID if depakote delayed release used	Partial, primary GTC, generalized seizures absence, JME, Lennox–Gastaut syndrome	GI upset, sedation, unsteadiness, tremor, thrombocytopenia, acute hepatic failure, hyperammonemia; alopecia, acute pancreatitis, polycystic ovary-like syndrome, weight gain, menstrual cycle irregularities
	Titration	Increase by 10 mg/kg/week		
	Maximum	60 mg/kg (3,000–5,000 mg) (TID); if depakote delayed release BID; if depakote XR used then QD		
Vigabatrin (Sabril)	Initial	1,000 mg/day (BID)	Infantile spasms, partial (refractory only)	CNS side effects, weight gain, tremor, anemia, permanent vision loss, peripheral neuropathy, abnormal MRI brain signal changes (in infants with infantile spasms)
	Titration	Increase by 500 mg every week		
	Maximum	3,000 mg/day (BID)		
Zonisamide (Zonegran)	Initial	100–200 mg/day (QD, higher dose give BID)	Partial, primary GTC, JME	Dizziness, cognitive impairment, nausea, sedation, rash, metabolic acidosis, oligohydrosis, kidney stones, weight loss
	Titration	Increase by 200 mg every 2 weeks		
	Maximum	600 mg/day (BID)		

*CNS side effects include sedation/fatigue, ataxia/unsteadiness, and dizziness.

TABLE 4.2.4 Pharmacokinetic Characteristics of Antiepileptic Drugs

Drug	Half-Life (Hours)	Time to Steady State (Days)	Elimination	Induces	Inhibits	Target Serum Concentration
CBZ	12M; 5–14Co	21–28 for complete autoinduction	CYP34A, CYP1A2, CYP2C8	CYP1A2, CYP2C, CYP3A, GT	None	4–12 µg/mL (17–51 µmol/L)
Ethosuximide	A60; C30	6–12	CYP3A4, 12–20% (renal)	None	None	40–100 µg/mL (282–708 µmol/L)
FBM	16–22	5–7	CYP3A4, CYP2E1, other, 50% (renal)	CYP3A4	CYP2C19, β-oxidation	30–60 µg/mL (126–252 µmol/L)
Gabapentin	5–40	1–2	Almost 100% (renal)	None	None	2–20 µg/mL (12–117 µmol/L)
LAC (Vimpat)	15	3	CYP2C19, 70% (renal)	None	None	Not defined
LTG	25.4M	3–15	GT, 10% (renal)	GT	None	4–20 µg/mL (16–78 µmol/L)
LEV	7–10	2	Undergoes nonhepatic hydrolysis, 66% (renal)	None	None	12–46 µg/mL (70–270 µmol/L)
Oxcarbazepine	3–13	2	Cytosolic system, 1% parent drug, 27% metabolite (renal)	CYP3A4, CYP3A5, GT	CYP2C19	3–35 µg/mL (MHD) (12–139 µmol/L)
PB	A46–136; C37–73	14–21	CYP2C9, other, 25% (renal)	CYP3A, CYP2C, GT	None	10–40 µg/mL (43–172 µmol/L)
PHT	A10–34; C5–14	7–28	CYP2C9, CYP2C19, 5% (renal)	CYP3A, CYP2C, GT	None	Total: 10–20 mg/mL (40–79 µmol/L) Unbound: 0.5–3 µg/mL (2–12 µmol/L)
Pregabalin (Lyrica)	A6–7	1–2	100% (renal)	None	None	Not defined

(Continued)

TABLE 4.2.4 Pharmacokinetic Characteristics of Antiepileptic Drugs (Continued)

Drug	Half-Life (Hours)	Time to Steady State (Days)	Elimination	Induces	Inhibits	Target Serum Concentration
PRM	A3.3–19; C4.5–14	1–4	Mostly renal, same as PB[a]	Same as PB[a]	None	5–10 µg/mL (23–46 µmol/L)
RUF (Banzel)	6–10	2	Hydrolysis, 2% (renal)	CYP3A4 (weak)	CYP2E1 (weak)	Not defined
TGB (Gabitril)	5–13	2	CYP3A4, 2% (renal)	None	None	0.02–0.2 µg/mL (0.05–0.5 µmol/L)
TPM	18–21	4–5	Hepatic enzymes not known; 70% (renal)	CYP3A4 (dose dependent)	CYP2C19	5–20 µg/mL (15–59 µmol/L)
Valproic acid	A8–20; C7–14	1–3	GT, β-oxidation, 2% (renal)	None	CYP2C9, GT, epoxide hydrolase	50–100 µg/mL (347–693 µmol/L)
Vigabatrin (Sabril)	5–8	N/A	Almost 100% (renal)	CYP2C9	None	0.8–36 µg/mL (6–279 µmol/L)
ZON	24–60	5–15	CYP3A4, 35% (renal)	None	None	10–40 µg/mL (47–188 µmol/L)

A, adult; C, child; Co, combination therapy; M, monotherapy; N/A, not applicable since effect depends on inhibiting enzyme.

Sources: (1) Faught E. Pharmacokinetic considerations in prescribing antiepileptic drugs. Epilepsia. 2001;42(Suppl 4):19–23. (2) Patsalos PN, Berry DJ, Bourgeois BFD, et al. Antiepileptic drugs—best practice guidelines for therapeutic drug monitoring: a position paper by the subcommission on therapeutic drug monitoring, ILAE Commission on Therapeutic Strategies. Epilepsia. 2008;49:1239–1276. (3) Halford JJ, Lapointe M. Clinical perspectives on lacosamide. Epilepsy Curr. 2009;9:1–9. (4) Sabril [product information]. Deerfield, IL: Lundbeck Inc; Feb 2012.

[a]Clinically relevant concentration of PB formed only when patient is on a hepatic enzyme inducer.

TABLE 4.2.5 Interactions Between Antiepileptic Drugs

AED	Added Drug	Effect	AED	Added Drug	Effect
CBZ	FBM	↑10,11 epoxide[a]	Pregabalin	No known interactions	
	Oxcarbazepine	↓CBZ	PRM	CBZ	↓PRM, ↑PB
	PB	↓CBZ		PHT	↓PRM, ↑PB
	PHT	↓CBZ		VPA	↑PRM, ↑PB
	Valproic acid (VPA)	↑10,11 epoxide[a]	RUF	CBZ	↓RUF
Ethosuximide	CBZ	↓Ethosuximide		PB	↓RUF
	PB	↓Ethosuximide		PHT	↓RUF
	PHT	↓Ethosuximide		PRM	↓RUF
				VPA	↑RUF
FBM	CBZ	↓FBM	TGB	CBZ	↓TGB
	PHT	↓FBM		PB	↓TGB
	VPA	↑FBM		PHT	↓TGB
				PRM	↓TGB
Gabapentin	No known interactions		TPM	CBZ	↓TPM
LAC	CBZ	↓LAC		PB	↓TPM
	PB	↓LAC		PHT	↓TPM
	PHT	↓LAC		PRM	↓TPM
LTG	CBZ	↓LTG		VPA	↓TPM
	PB	↓LTG			
	PHT	↓LTG			
	PRM	↓LTG			
	VPA	↑LTG			

(Continued)

TABLE 4.2.5 Interactions Between Antiepileptic Drugs (Continued)

AED	Added Drug	Effect	AED	Added Drug	Effect
LEV	CBZ	↓LEV	VPA	CBZ	↓VPA
	PB	↓LEV		FBM	↑VPA
	PHT	↓LEV		LTG	↓VPA
Oxcarbazepine[b]	CBZ	↓MHD		PB	↓VPA
	PB	↓MHD		PHT	↓VPA
	PHT	↓MHD		PRM	↓VPA
PB	FBM	↑PB		TPM	↓VPA
	Oxcarbazepine	↑PB	Vigabatrin	No known interactions	
	PHT	↑PB	ZON	CBZ	↓ZON
	VPA	↑PB		PB	↓ZON
PHT	CBZ	↑ or ↓PHT		PHT	↓ZON
	FBM	↑PHT		PRM	↓ZON
	Methsuximide	↑PHT			
	Oxcarbazepine (>1200 mg/d)	↑PHT			
	PB	↑ or ↓PHT			
	TPM	↑PHT			
	VPA	↓PHT, then may ↑PHT			
	Vigabatrin	↓PHT			

Reproduced with permission from Rogers SJ, Cavazos JE. Epilepsy. In: Dipiro JT, Talbert RL, Yee GC, Matzke GR, Wells BG, Posey LM, eds. *Pharmacotherapy: A Pathophysiologic Approach.* 8th ed. New York, NY: McGraw-Hill Companies; 2011.

[a]Carbamazepine-10,11-epoxide is an active metabolite of CBZ.

[b]Oxcarbazepine is a prodrug that is converted to the active 10-monohydroxy derivative (10 MHD) by glucuronidation.

FIGURE 4.3.1 Diagnostic Criteria for Parkinson's Disease

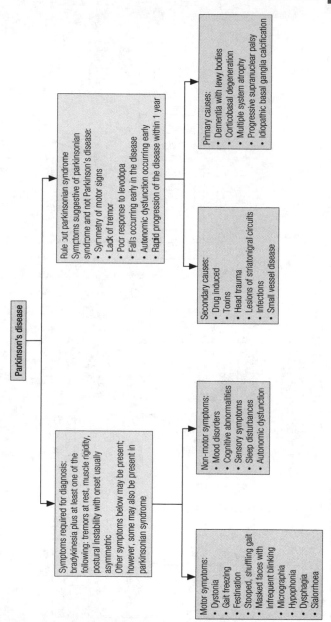

Source: Chen JJ, Lew MF, Siderowf A. Treatment strategies and quality-of-care indicators for patients with Parkinson's disease. *JMCP.* 2009;15(3):S1–S21.

FIGURE 4.3.2 Pharmacotherapy of Early Parkinson's Disease

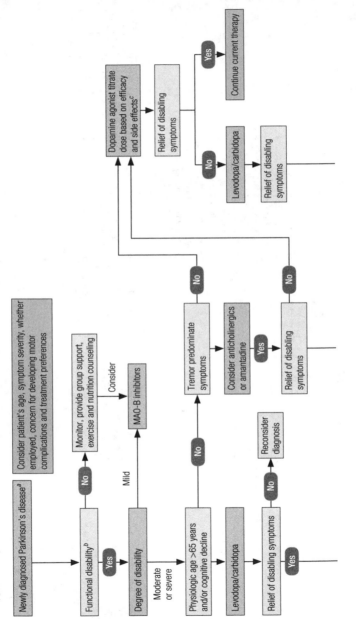

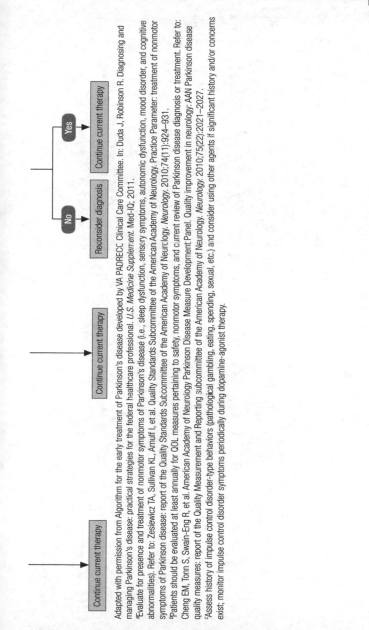

Adapted with permission from Algorithm for the early treatment of Parkinson's disease developed by VA PADRECC Clinical Care Committee. In: Duda J, Robinson R. Diagnosing and managing Parkinson's disease: practical strategies for the federal healthcare professional. *U.S. Medicine Supplement.* Med-IQ; 2011.

[a]Evaluate for presence and treatment of nonmotor symptoms of Parkinson's disease (i.e., sleep dysfunction, sensory symptoms, autonomic dysfunction, mood disorder, and cognitive abnormalities). Refer to: Zesiewicz TA, Sullivan KL, Arnulf I, et al. Quality Standards Subcommittee of the American Academy of Neurology. Practice Parameter: treatment of nonmotor symptoms of Parkinson disease: report of the Quality Standards Subcommittee of the American Academy of Neurology. *Neurology.* 2010;74(11):924–931.

[b]Patients should be evaluated at least annually for QOL measures pertaining to safety, nonmotor symptoms, and current review of Parkinson disease diagnosis or treatment. Refer to: Cheng EM, Tonn S, Swain-Eng R, et al. American Academy of Neurology Parkinson Disease Measure Development Panel. Quality improvement in neurology: AAN Parkinson disease quality measures: report of the Quality Measurement and Reporting subcommittee of the American Academy of Neurology. *Neurology.* 2010;75(22):2021–2027.

[c]Assess history of impulse control disorder-type behaviors (pathological gambling, eating, spending, sexual, etc.) and consider using other agents if significant history and/or concerns exist; monitor impulse control disorder symptoms periodically during dopamine-agonist therapy.

FIGURE 4.3.3 Management of Motor Complications in Parkinson's Disease

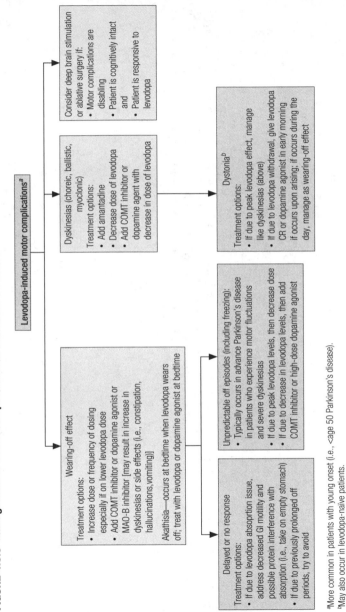

Levodopa-induced motor complications[a]

Consider deep brain stimulation or ablative surgery if:
- Motor complications are disabling
- Patient is cognitively intact and
- Patient is responsive to levodopa

Dyskinesias (choreic, ballistic, myoclonic)
Treatment options:
- Add amantadine
- Decrease dose of levodopa
- Add COMT inhibitor or dopamine agent with decrease in dose of levodopa

Dystonia[b]
Treatment options:
- If due to peak levodopa effect, manage like dyskinesias (above)
- If due to levodopa withdrawal, give levodopa CR or dopamine agonist in early morning
- If occurs upon arising; if occurs during the day, manage as wearing-off effect

Wearing-off effect
Treatment options:
- Increase dose or frequency of dosing especially if on lower levodopa dose
- Add COMT inhibitor or dopamine agonist or MAO-B inhibitor [may result in increase in dyskinesias or side effects (i.e., constipation, hallucinations, vomiting)]
Akathisia—occurs at bedtime when levodopa wears off; treat with levodopa or dopamine agonist at bedtime

Unpredictable off episodes (including freezing):
- Typically occurs in advance Parkinson's disease in patients who experience motor fluctuations and severe dyskinesias
- If due to peak levodopa levels, then decrease dose
- If due to decrease in levodopa levels, then add COMT inhibitor or high-dose dopamine agonist

Delayed or no response
Treatment options:
- If due to levodopa absorption issue, address decreased GI motility and possible protein interference with absorption (i.e., take on empty stomach)
- If due to previously prolonged off periods, try to avoid

[a]More common in patients with young onset (i.e., <age 50 Parkinson's disease).
[b]May also occur in levodopa-naïve patients.

TABLE 4.3.4 Considerations for Anti-Parkinson's Agents

Therapy	Comments
Dopamine agonists	As a class associated with nausea, vomiting, confusion, hallucinations, postural hypotension, lower-extremity edema, vivid dreaming and less commonly compulsive behaviors (hypersexuality, gambling, Internet use, hoarding, shopping), and sleep attacks; are ineffective in patients who do not respond to levodopa; avoid stopping abruptly due to possible dopamine withdrawal syndrome associated with symptoms of anxiety, panic attacks, depression, sweating, nausea, fatigue, dizziness, pain; levodopa does not treat this withdrawal
Dopamine replacement	Common side effects are nausea, vomiting, orthostasis, hallucinations, dyskinesias, and wearing- off motor fluctuations
Monamine oxidase type B inhibitors	Use of these agents contraindicated in patients taking meperidine and other selected opioid analgesics due to risk of serotonin syndrome; not contraindicated in patients on serotonin reuptake in ibitor antidepressants; higher doses are more likely to have some MAO-A inhibitory activity
Anticholinergics	Class of drugs causes dry mouth, blurred vision, constipation, urinary retention, confusion, hallucinations, sedation with associated increased risk of falls and memory impairment; avoid stopping these drugs abruptly due to withdrawal symptoms; tolerated better in young, cognitively intact patients; for treatment of tremor or dystonia

TABLE 4.3.5 Drug Products and Dosing in Parkinson's Disease

Medications	Daily Dose	Comments
Dopamine Agonists		
Apomorphine injection 10 mg/mL	Initial 2 mg subcutaneous test dose, then 1 mg less than tolerated test dose; increase by 1 mg every few days; maintenance dose 2–6 mg divided 3 times/day; rotate injection sites to avoid developing subcutaneous nodules	Premedicate 3 days before with trimethobenzamide due to nausea and vomiting; use contraindicated with serotonin receptor blocker class drugs due to severe hypotension and syncope; avoid prochlorperazine and metoclopramide since they reduce apomorphine's effectiveness
Bromocriptine tablet, capsule	Initial dose 1.25 mg/day; increase slowly over 4–6 weeks; maintenance dose 10–40 mg divided 3 times/day	Ergot-derived agonist with possible associated side effect, rarely cardiovascular valve fibrosis, Raynaud phenomenon, erythromelalgia, retroperitoneal/pulmonary fibrosis
Pramipexole tablet[a]	0.125 mg 3 times/day; titrate weekly by 0.125–0.25 mg/dose; maintenance dose 1.5–4.5 mg divided 3 times/day	Renally excreted; adjust dose function in renally impaired patient
Ropinirole tablet[a]	0.25 mg 3 times/day; titrate weekly by 0.25 mg/dose	Metabolized by CYP1A2 therefore potent inhibitors (i.e., fluoroquinolone antibiotics) and inducers (i.e., cigarette smoking) may change serum levels of this drug
Carbidopa/Levodopa tablet[a]	25/100 once/day (regular or oral disintegrating tablet); increase by 25/100 weekly to desired effect and as tolerated; maintenance dose is 30/300–150/1500 in divided doses given 3–5 times/day	Avoid high-protein meals; take regular release product 60 minutes before meals; take controlled release product with food
	25/100 2 times/day (controlled release tablet); space at least 6 hours apart and increase every 3–7 days; maintenance dose is 50/200–500/2,000 divided 4 times/day	Controlled release product is not very effective for managing levodopa-induced motor fluctuations
COMT Inhibitors		
Entacapone tablet	One tablet with each administration of levodopa/carbidopa up to 8 tablets daily; maintenance dose is 3–8 tablets/day	Diarrhea 10% patients—occurs 6–12 weeks after starting drug; can cause urine discoloration

Drug	Dosing	Comments
Entacapone/levodopa/carbidopa combination tablet		Use only after stabilized on dose of levodopa/carbidopa
Tolcapone tablet	100–200 mg 3 times/day; maintenance dose is 300–600 mg divided 3 times/day	More effective than entacapone; can cause fatal liver failure especially first 6 months; need frequent liver enzyme testing; diarrhea 10% patients—occurs 6–12 weeks after starting drug
Monoamine Oxidase Type B Inhibitors		
Selegiline tablet, capsule, oral disintegrating tablet, transdermal patch[b]	5 mg/day; may increase to 5 mg 2 times/day; maintenance dose oral tablet is 5–10 mg/day given as 5 mg with breakfast and 5 mg with lunch. Oral disintegrating tablet maintenance dose is 1.25–2.5 mg/day	Hepatically metabolized to l-methamphetamine and l-amphetamine; side effects can include insomnia, jitteriness, and hallucinations; increases peak affects of l-dopa and can worsen preexisting dyskinesias or psychiatric symptoms; oral disintegrating tablet less likely to cause above effects since product avoids first-pass hepatic metabolism with decreased production of amphetamine metabolites
Rasagiline tablet	0.5 mg/day; may increase to 1 mg/day; maintenance dose is 0.5–1 mg/day	Drug not metabolized to amphetamine metabolites; metabolized by CYP1A2; studies indicate probably more effective than selegiline as adjunctive agent
Anticholinergics		
Benztropine tablet	0.5 mg/day; increased by 0.5 mg every 3–5 days; maintenance dose is 1–3 mg 1–2 times/day	
Trihexyphenidyl tablet, liquid	1–2 mg/day increased by 1–2 mg every 3–5 days; maintenance dose is 6–15 mg 2–3 times/day	
Miscellaneous Agent		
Amantadine tablet, capsule, liquid	100 mg/day; increased by 100 mg every 1–2 weeks; maintenance dose is 100–300 mg/day; avoid giving near bedtime	Renally excreted; adjust dose in renally impaired patients; can cause confusion, nightmares, insomnia, hallucinations, irritability, and livedo reticularis. Modest symptomatic treatment of tremor, rigidity and bradykinesia

[a]Sustained-release formulation available.
[b]Transdermal patch not FDA approved for treatment of Parkinson's disease.

FIGURE 4.4.1 Diagnostic Criteria for Episodic Headaches

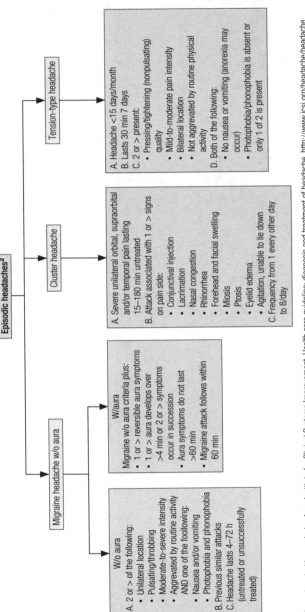

Reproduced with permission from Institute for Clinical Systems Improvement. Health care guideline: diagnosis and treatment of headache. http://www.icsi.org/headache/headache_diagnosis_and_treatment_of_2609.html. January 2011. Accessed June 2, 2011.
^aRule out organic disorder by evaluation and diagnostic studies in workup.

Episodic headaches^a

Migraine headache w/o aura

W/o aura
A. 2 or > of the following:
• Unilateral location
• Pulsating/throbbing
• Moderate-to-severe intensity
• Aggravated by routine activity
AND one of the following:
• Nausea and/or vomiting
• Photophobia and phonophobia
B. Previous similar attacks
C. Headache lasts 4–72 h (untreated or unsuccessfully treated)

W/aura
Migraine w/o aura criteria plus:
• 1 or > reversible aura symptoms
• 1 or > aura develops over >4 min or 2 or > symptoms occur in succession
• Aura symptoms do not last >60 min
• Migraine attack follows within 60 min

Cluster headache

A. Severe unilateral orbital, supraorbital and/or temporal pain lasting 15–180 min untreated
B. Attack associated with 1 or > signs on pain side:
• Conjunctival injection
• Lacrimation
• Nasal congestion
• Rhinorrhea
• Forehead and facial swelling
• Miosis
• Ptosis
• Eyelid edema
• Agitation, unable to lie down
C. Frequency from 1 every other day to 8/day

Tension-type headache

A. Headache <15 days/month
B. Lasts 30 min 7 days
C. 2 or > present:
• Pressing/tightening (nonpulsating) quality
• Mild-to-moderate pain intensity
• Bilateral location
• Not aggravated by routine physical activity
D. Both of the following:
• No nausea or vomiting (anorexia may occur)
• Photophobia/phonophobia is absent or only 1 of 2 is present

FIGURE 4.4.2 Pharmacotherapy of Episodic Headaches

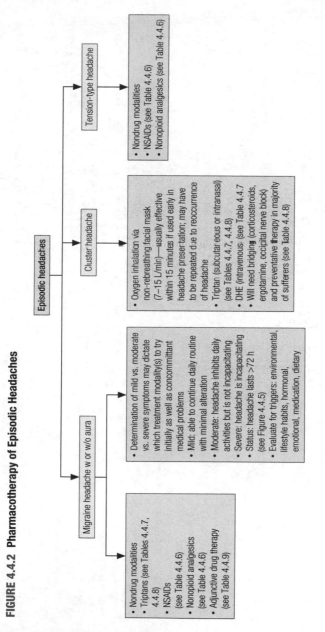

Episodic headaches

Migraine headache w or w/o aura

- Determination of mild vs. moderate vs. severe symptoms may dictate which treatment modality(s) to try initially as well as concommittant medical problems
- Mild: able to continue daily routine with minimal alteration
- Moderate: headache inhibits daily activities but is not incapacitating
- Severe: headache is incapacitating
- Status: headache lasts >72 h (see Figure 4.4.5)
- Evaluate for triggers: environmental, lifestyle habits, hormonal, emotional, medication, dietary

Nondrug modalities
- Triptans (see Tables 4.4.7, 4.4.8)
- NSAIDs (see Table 4.4.6)
- Nonopioid analgesics (see Table 4.4.6)
- Adjunctive drug therapy (see Table 4.4.9)

Cluster headache

- Oxygen inhalation via non-rebreathing facial mask (7–15 L/min)—usually effective within 15 minutes if used early in headache presentation; may have to be repeated due to reoccurrence of headache
- Triptan (subcutaneous or intranasal) (see Tables 4.4.7, 4.4.8)
- DHE (intravenous) (see Table 4.4.7)
- Will need bridging (corticosteroids, ergotamine, occipital nerve block) and preventative therapy in majority of sufferers (see Table 4.4.8)

Tension-type headache

- Nondrug modalities (see Table 4.4.6)
- NSAIDs (see Table 4.4.6)
- Nonopioid analgesics (see Table 4.4.6)

FIGURE 4.4.3 Diagnostic Criteria for Chronic Headaches.

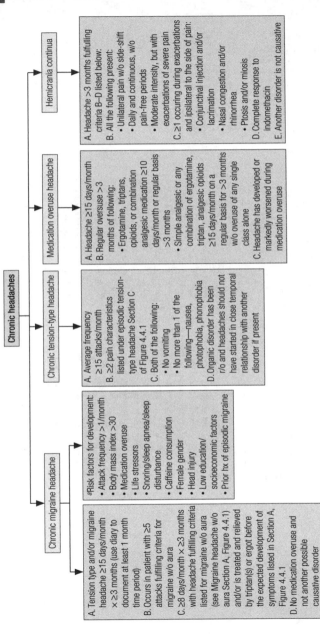

Reproduced with permission from Institute for Clinical Systems Improvement. Health care guideline: diagnosis and treatment of headache. http://www.icsi.org/headache/headache_diagnosis_and_treatment_of_2609.html. January 2011. Accessed June 3, 2011.
[a]*Neurology: Clinical Practice* 2011;76(suppl2):S37-S42

FIGURE 4.4.4 Pharmacotherapy of Chronic Headaches

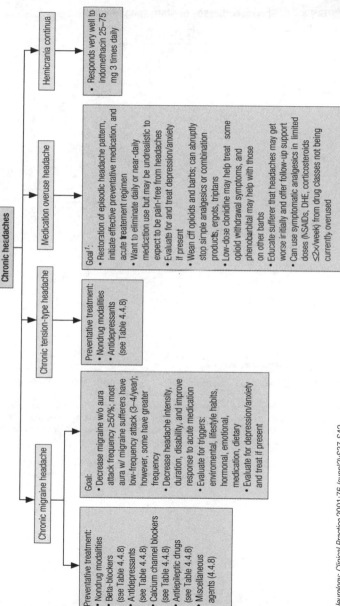

Chronic headaches

Chronic migraine headache

Preventative treatment:
- Nondrug modalities
- Beta-blockers (see Table 4.4.8)
- Antidepressants (see Table 4.4.8)
- Calcium channel blockers (see Table 4.4.8)
- Antiepileptic drugs (see Table 4.4.8)
- Miscellaneous agents (4.4.8)

Goal:
- Decrease migraine w/o aura attack frequency ≥50%; most aura w/ migraine sufferers have low-frequency attack (3–4/year); however, some have greater frequency
- Decrease headache intensity, duration, disability, and improve response to acute medication
- Evaluate for triggers: environmental, lifestyle habits, hormonal, emotional, medication, dietary
- Evaluate for depression/anxiety and treat if present

Chronic tension-type headache

Preventative treatment:
- Nondrug modalities
- Antidepressants (see Table 4.4.8)

Medication overuse headache

Goal[1]:
- Restoration of episodic headache pattern, initiate effective preventative medication, and acute treatment regimen
- Want to eliminate daily or near-daily medication use but may be undealistic to expect to be pain-free from headaches
- Evaluate for and treat depression/anxiety if present
- Wean off opioids and barbs; can abruptly stop simple analgesics or combination products, ergots, triptans
- Low-dose clonidine may help treat some opioid withdrawal symptoms, and phenobarbital may help with those on other barbs
- Educate sufferer that headaches may get worse initially and offer follow-up support
- Can use symptomatic analgesics in limited doses (NSAIDs, DHE, corticosteroids ≤2×/week) from drug classes not being currently overused

Hemicrania continua

- Responds very well to indomethacin 25–75 mg 3 times daily

[1]*Neurology: Clinical Practice* 2001;76 (suppl2):S37–S42

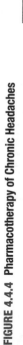

FIGURE 4.4.5 Pharmacotherapy of Status Migrainosus

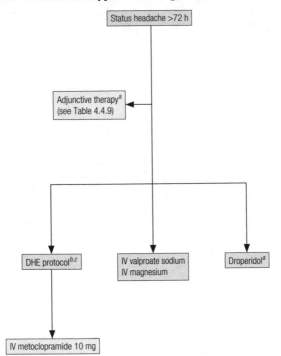

[a]Patient should be hydrated prior to neuroleptic treatment with 250–500 mL fluid to avoid orthostatic hypotension.

[b]Avoid in a pregnant patient or who has a history of heart disease or Prinzmetal's angina, severe peripheral vascular disease, onset of chest pain following test dose of DHE, within 24 hours of receiving a triptan or ergot derivative, elevated blood pressure, cerebrovascular disease, patients with hemiplegic or basilar-type migraines (defined as any three of the following: diplopia, dysarthria, tinnitus, vertigo, transient hearing loss, or mental confusion)

[c]See Institute for Clinical Systems Improvement. Health care guideline: diagnosis and treatment of headache. http://www.icsi.org/headache/headache_diagnosis_and_treatment_of_2609.html.January2011.

TABLE 4.4.6 Nonsteroidal Anti-Inflammatory Drugs and Non-Opioid Analgesics for Headache

Drug	Daily Dose	Comments
NSAIDs		
Aspirin	500–1,000 mg every 4–6 hours	Maximum daily dose 4 g
Ibuprofen	200–800 mg every 6 hours	Avoid doses >2.4 g/day
Naproxen sodium	550–825 mg at onset, can repeat 220 mg in 3–4 hours	Avoid doses >1,375 g/day
Naproxen 500 mg/ sumatriptan 85 mg	1 tablet at onset, can repeat 1 tablet in 2 hours; maximum daily dose 2 tablets	Do not crush or chew tablets
Diclofenac potassium	50–100 mg at onset; can repeat 50 mg in 8 hours	Avoid doses >150 mg/day
Ketorolac nasal spray	1 spray in each nostril every 6–8 hours; maximum daily dose 126 mg	Dose decreased to 1 spray in only 1 nostril in patient ≥65 years old, renally impaired, or <50 kg; maximum daily dose 63 mg

Nasal spray should be discarded within 24 hours after using the first dose |
| Ketorolac injection | 30 mg IV; 60 mg IM; can repeat dose in 6 hours; maximum daily dose 120 mg | Dose decreased to 15 mg IV; 30 mg IM in patients with criteria listed above; can repeat dose in 6 hours; maximum daily dose 60 mg

Oral form is indicated only for continuation of injectable treatment up to 5 days total |
Non-opioid Analgesics		
Acetaminophen	1,000 mg at onset; repeat every 4–6 hours as needed	Maximum daily dose is 4 g
Acetaminophen 250 mg/ aspirin 250 mg/caffeine 65 mg	1–2 tablets every 4–6 hours	Available over-the-counter as Excedrin Migraine
Aspirin or acetaminophen with butalbital, caffeine	1–2 tablets every 4–6 hours	Limit dose to 4 tablets/day and usage to 2 days/week due to increase risk of developing chronic headache
Butorphanol nasal spray	1 spray in 1 nostril at onset, may repeat in 1 hour	Limited to 4 sprays/day; use when non-opioid therapies not effective or not tolerated
Lidocaine nasal solution (4%)	1–4 drops in 1 nostril at onset of headache (both nostrils if headache is bilateral)	Pain relief within 15 minutes but recurrence is common; for cluster headaches use phenylephrine drops 0.5% before lidocaine to facilitate decongestion

TABLE 4.4.7   Serotonin Agonists (Triptans) and Ergotamine Products[b]

Drug	Dose	Comments
Triptans[a]		
Almotriptan tablets	6.25 or 12.5 mg at onset; may repeat in 2 hours	Optimal dose 12.5 mg; maximum dose 25 mg
		Significant efficacy over placebo in 12–17 years olds
Eletriptan tablets	20 or 40 mg at onset; may repeat in 2 hours	Maximum single dose 40 mg; maximum daily dose 80 mg
Frovatriptan tablets	2.5 or 5 mg at onset; may repeat in 2 hours	Optimal dose 2.5–5 mg; maximum daily dose 7.5 mg
Naratriptan tablets	1 or 2.5 mg at onset; may repeat in 4 hours	Optimal dose 2.5 mg; maximum daily dose 5 mg
Rizatriptan tablets	5 or 10 mg at onset (regular or oral disintegrating tablet); may repeat in 2 hours	Optimal dose is 10 mg; maximum daily dose 30 mg; onset of effect similar with two oral dosage forms; use lower dose (5 mg) in patients on propranolol with maximum daily dose 15 mg; do not give within 2 weeks of an MOAI
Sumatriptan tablets	25, 50, 85, or 100 mg at onset; may repeat in 2 hours	Optimal dose 50–100 mg; maximum dose 200 mg/day; combination product with naproxen, 85 mg/ 500 mg; do not give within 2 weeks of an MOAI
Sumatriptan nasal spray	5, 10, or 20 mg at onset; may repeat in 2 hours	Optimal dose 20 mg; maximum daily dose 40 mg; single-dose device delivers 5 or 20 mg; use 1 spray in 1 nostril; do not give within 2 weeks of an MOAI
Sumatriptan injection	6 mg subcutaneously at onset; may repeat in 1 hour	Maximum daily dose 12 mg; do not give within 2 weeks of an MOAI
Zolmitriptan tablets	2.5 or 5 mg at onset (regular or disintegrating tablet); may repeat in 2 hours	Optimal dose 2.5 mg; maximum daily dose 10 mg; do not divide disintegrating tablet; do not give within 2 weeks of an MOAI
Zolmitriptan nasal spray	5 mg (1 spray) at onset; may repeat in 2 hours	Maximum daily dose 10 mg; do not give within 2 weeks of an MOAI

Ergotamine Products[b]		
DHE nasal spray	1 spray (0.5 mg) in each nostril at onset; repeat 15 minutes later (total 4 sprays)	Maximum daily dose 3 mg; prime sprayer 4 times before using; do not tilt head back or inhale through nose while spraying; discard open ampules after 8 hours
DHE injection 1 mg/mL	0.25–1 mg at onset IM, IV, or subcutaneously; may repeat every hour	Maximum daily dose 3 mg or 6 mg/week
Ergotamine tartrate oral tablet (1 mg) w/ caffeine 100 mg	2 mg at onset; then 1–2 mg every 30 minutes as needed	Maximum daily dose 6 mg or 10 mg/week; consider pretreatment with antiemetic
Ergotamine tartrate sublingual tablet (2 mg)	Same as above for oral tablet	Same as above for oral tablet
Ergotamine tartrate rectal suppository (2 mg) with caffeine (100 mg)	Insert ½ to 1 suppository at onset; may repeat after 1 hour	Maximum daily dose 4 mg or 10 mg/week; consider pretreatment with an antiemetic

Reproduced with permission from Minor DS. Headache disorders. In: Dipro JT, Talbert RL, Yee GC, Matzke GR, Wells BG, Posey LM, eds. *Pharmacotherapy. A Pathophysiologic Approach.* 8th ed. New York, NY: McGraw-Hill Companies; 2011.

[a]Large intersubject variability in response; efficacy is higher and more complete if used early when headache is of mild intensity; should not be given within 24 hours of an ergotamine derivative; contraindicated in patients with ischemic heart disease, uncontrolled hypertension, cerebrovascular disease, hemiplegic, and basilar migraine.
[b]Contraindicated in patients with renal or hepatic disease, coronary, cerebral, or peripheral vascular disease, uncontrolled hypertension, sepsis, and in women who are pregnant or nursing.

TABLE 4.4.8 Other Preventative Drug Therapies

Drug	Daily Dose	Comments
Beta Blockers		
Propranolol[a,b]	80–240 mg	• First-line therapy
Timolol[a]	10–20 mg	• Can exacerbate asthma, second- or third-degree heart block, left ventricular dysfunction, peripheral vascular disease, and impair physical activity
Metoprolol[b]	50–200 mg	
Atenolol	50–100 mg	• May see increased efficacy in some patients if used with TCA (can use lower dose of TCA)
Nadolol	80–120 mg	
Nebivolol	5 mg	
Antiepileptics		
TPM[a]	50–200 mg	• First-line therapy (except gabapentin)
VPA/divalproex[a,b]	800–1,000 mg	• TPM side effects: paresthesias, weight loss, taste disturbance, memory problems, renal stones
Gabapentin	1,200–2,400 mg	• VPA side effects: nausea, fatigue, tremor, weight gain, dizziness, birth defects
LTG	100 mg	• Gabapentin side effects: sedation, dizziness, weight gain
		• Titrate LTG dose up slowly by 25 mg every 2 weeks to avoid skin rash; has been effective only in migraine with aura
Antidepressants		
Amitriptyline	25–150 mg	• First-line therapy (TCA efficacy increases with duration of treatment; more likely to reduce intensity of migraine) (*Neurol Sci.* 2011;32:S1111)
Nortriptyline	10–150 mg	
Desipramine	150 mg	
Doxepin	10–300 mg	• Avoid in patients intolerant of anticholinergic effects (dry mouth and eyes, constipation, urinary retention, confusion, cardiac effects)
Venlafaxine[b]	75–225 mg	
Calcium Channel Blocker		
Verapamil[b]	240–480 mg	• Second-line therapy
		• Avoid in patients with second- or third-degree heart block or left ventricular dysfunction
Angiotensin-Converting Enzyme Inhibitor		
Lisinopril	20 mg	• Second- or third-line therapy
		• Avoid in patients at risk for angioedema, renal insufficiency, hypotension, volume depletion, hyperkalemia, and pregnant patients
Angiotensin II Receptor Blocker		
Candesartan	16 mg	• Second- or third-line therapy
		• Same as lisinopril above except angioedema
Botulinum Toxin		
OnabotulinumtoxinA (Botox©)[a]	155 units divided in 31 sites (head and neck)	Does not help episodic migraine; repeat in 12 weeks

TABLE 4.4.8 Other Preventative Drug Therapies *(Continued)*

Drug	Daily Dose	Comments
Herbal Agents, Vitamins, Minerals		
Coenzyme Q10	300 mg	Divide dose to avoid GI upset; decreases frequency of migraine; may take up to 3 months to work; useful in treatment of migraine in children
Petasites hybridus extract (butterbur root) (Petadolex©)	150 mg	Divide dose to avoid GI upset; avoid in patient allergic to daisies; may decrease frequency of migraine in children (preliminary evidence)
Feverfew	250 μg	Dose refers to active ingredient parthenolide; avoid in patient allergic to daises; avoid in pregnant patient since may cause uterus to contract
Riboflavin (vitamin B$_2$)	400 mg	Decreases frequency of migraine
Magnesium	400–600 mg (different salts)	Appropriate choice for women who are pregnant or trying to conceive; especially for migraine with aura; oxide salt shown to be useful in children to decrease frequency and severity of migraine

[a]FDA approved.
[b]Sustained-release formulation available.

TABLE 4.4.9 Adjunctive Drug Therapies for Headaches

Drug	Dose	Comments
Caffeine	Minimal 65 mg orally	Can cause tremor, nausea
Metoclopramide	10 mg IV at onset	Can cause drowsiness, extrapyramidal symptoms
Prochlorperazine	5–10 mg IV, IM, or 25 mg suppository rectally	
Promethazine	25 mg IV, IM or suppository rectally	

Reproduced with permission from Institute for Clinical Systems Improvement. Health care guideline: diagnosis and treatment of headache. http://www.icsi.org/headache/headache_diagnosis_and_treatment_of_2609.html. January 2011. Accessed June 3, 2011.

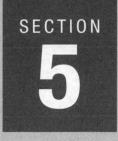

ABBREVIATIONS

ANV	Anticipatory nausea and vomiting	NK-1	Neurokinin 1
CINV	Chemotherapy-induced nausea and vomiting	NSAID	Nonsteroidal anti-inflammatory drug
		PONV	Postoperative nausea and vomiting
COX-2	Cyclooxygenase-2	PPI	Proton pump inhibitor
GERD	Gastroesophageal reflux disease	PUD	Peptic ulcer disease
5-HT3	5-Hydroxytryptamine-3	RINV	Radiation-induced nausea and vomiting
H_2RA	Histamine 2 receptor antagonist		
MALT	Mucosa-associated lymphoid tissue		

TABLE 5.1.1 Drugs for Treatment of Nausea and Vomiting

Drug	Typical Dosing	Dosage Forms
Antihistaminic/Anticholinergic Agents[a]		
Cyclizine (Marezine)	50 mg before travel; may repeat in 4–6 h PRN	Tab
Dimenhydrinate (Dramamine)	50–100 mg Q 4–6 h PRN	Tab, chew tab, cap
Diphenhydramine (Benadryl)	25–50 mg Q 4–6 h PRN	Tab, cap, liquid
	10–50 mg Q 2–4 h PRN	IM, IV
Hydroxyzine (Vistaril, Atarax)	25–100 mg Q 4–6 h PRN	IM (unlabeled use)
Meclizine (Antivert)	12.5–25 mg 1 h before travel; repeat Q 12–24 h PRN	Tab, chew tab
Scopolamine (Transderm Scop)	1.5 mg Q 72 h	Transdermal patch
Trimethobenzamide (Tigan)	300 mg TID-QID	Cap
Benzodiazepines[b]		
Alprazolam (Xanax)	0.5–2 mg TID	Tab
Lorazepam (Ativan)	0.5–1 mg TID	Tab, IV
Dopamine-2 Receptor Antagonists		
Chlorpromazine (Thorazine)	10–25 mg Q 4–6 h PRN	Tab, liquid
	25–50 mg Q 4–6 h PRN	IM, IV
Droperidol (Inapsine)	2.5 mg; additional 1.25 mg may be given	IM, IV
Haloperidol (Haldol)	1–5 mg Q 12 h PRN	Tab, liquid, IM, IV
Metoclopramide (Reglan)	10 mg QID (before meals and at bedtime)	Tab, IV
	20–40 mg TID-QID	Tab, IV
Prochlorperazine (Compazine)	5–10 mg 3–4 QD PRN	Tab, liquid
	5–10 mg Q 3–4 h PRN	IM
	2.5–10 mg Q 3–4 h PRN	IV
	25 mg BID PRN	Supp
Promethazine (Phenergan)	12.5–25 mg Q 4–6 h PRN	Tab, liquid, supp, IM[c]
5-HT3 Receptor Antagonists		
Ondansetron (Zofran)	4–8 mg BID-TID	Tab, ODT, IV

[a]Best used for vestibular nausea and vomiting.
[b]Weak antiemetics, useful as adjuncts or for anxiety-related nausea and vomiting.
[c]Avoid giving IV due to risk of severe extravasation injury.

TABLE 5.1.2 Drugs and Dosing for Prophylaxis of CINV and RINV

Drug	Indication	Dosing	Dosage Forms
5-HT3 Receptor Antagonists			
Dolasetron (Anzemet)	CINV	100 mg before chemo	Tab
	Delayed CINV	100 mg QD	Tab
Granisetron (Kytril)	CINV, RINV	2 mg before chemo/radiation	Tab
	Delayed CINV	1–2 mg QD	Tab
	CINV	1 mg before chemo	IV
	CINV	34.3 mg applied 24 h prior to chemo	Transdermal patch
Ondansetron (Zofran)	CINV	16-24 mg before chemo	Tab, ODT
	CINV	8–12 mg before chemo/radiation	IV
	RINV	8 mg BID	Tab, ODT
	Delayed CINV	8 mg QD-BID	Tab, ODT
Palonosetron (Aloxi)	CINV	0.25 mg before chemo	IV
	CINV	0.5 mg before chemo	Tab
NK-1 Receptor Antagonist			
Aprepitant (Emend)	CINV	125 mg before chemo	Cap
	Delayed CINV	80 mg days 2 and 3 after chemo	Cap
Fosaprepitant (Emend)	CINV	150 mg before chemo	IV
Benzodiazepines			
Alprazolam (Xanax)	ANV	0.5–2 mg TID prior to chemotherapy	Tab
Lorazepam (Ativan)	ANV	0.5–2 mg on night before and morning of chemotherapy	Tab
Corticosteroid			
Dexamethasone (Decadron)	CINV	8–12 mg before chemo[a]	Tab, IV
	Delayed CINV	8 mg QD days 2 and 3 after chemo	Tab, IV
	RINV	4 mg with fractions 1–5	Tab, IV

Sources: (1) Prevention of chemotherapy and radiotherapy-induced emesis. Results of the 2004 Perugia International Antiemetic Consensus Conference. *Ann Oncol*. 2006;17:20–28. (2) Basch E, Prestrud AA, Hesketh PJ, et al. Antiemetics: American Society of Clinical Oncology Clinical Practice Guideline Update. *J Clin Oncol*. 2011;29:4189–4198.

[a]12 mg for high emetic risk regimens or for moderate risk regimens including an NK1 antagonist, 8 mg for all other regimens.

TABLE 5.1.3 Regimens for Prophylaxis of CINV and RINV

Emetic Risk	Risk Definition	Regimen
CINV Regimens		
High	Anthracycline + cyclophosphamide, carmustine, cisplatin, cyclophosphamide ≥1500 mg/m², dacarbazine, dactinomycin, mechlorethamine, streptozotocin	5-HT3 antagonist (day 1) + dexamethasone (days 1–3)[a] + NK1 antagonist[b]
Moderate	Carboplatin, cytarabine >1 g/m², cyclophosphamide <1500 mg/m², daunorubicin, doxorubicin, epirubicin, idarubicin, ifosfamide, irinotecan, oxaliplatin, procarbazine	Preferred: Palonosetron (day 1) + dexamethasone (days 1–3) Alternative: 5-HT3 antagonist[c] + dexamethasone +/– NK1 antagonist
Low	Bortezomib, capecitabine, cetuximab, cytarabine >1 g/m², docetaxel, erlotinib, etoposide, fluorouracil, gemcitabine, lapatinib, methotrexate, mitomycin, mitoxantrone, paclitaxel, pemetrexed, sorafenib, sunitinib, temozolomide, topotecan, trastuzumab	Dexamethasone (day 1 only)
Delayed CINV		5-HT3 antagonist + dexamethasone +/– NK1 antagonist for 2–3 days after chemo
RINV Regimens		
Moderate to high	Upper abdomen, upper body, half body, or total body irradiation	5-HT3 antagonist (ondansetron or granisetron) before each fraction and 24 h after + dexamethasone for 5 days (fractions 1–5)
Low	Head, head and neck, lower thorax, pelvis	5-HT3 antagonist (ondansetron or granisetron) before each fraction

Sources: (1) Prevention of chemotherapy and radiotherapy-induced emesis. Results of the 2004 Perugia International Antiemetic Consensus Conference. *Ann Oncol.* 2006;17:20–28. (2) Basch E, Prestrud AA, Hesketh PJ, et al. Antiemetics: American Society of Clinical Oncology Clinical Practice Guideline Update. *J Clin Oncol.* 2011;29:4189–198.

[a]May also give dexamethasone on days 1–4.
[b]Days 1–3 for aprepitant, day 1 only for fosaprepitant.
[c]Ondansetron or granisetron preferred, unless an NK-1 antagonist is used.

TABLE 5.2.1 Recommendations for Evaluation and Treatment of GERD

Evaluation	Lifestyle Modifications[a]	Pharmacotherapy
• AGA GERD definition: "a condition which develops when the reflux of stomach contents causes troublesome symptoms and/or complications." Symptoms are "troublesome" if they adversely affect an individual's well-being.[a]	• Weight loss for obese or overweight patients • Elevation of the bed for patients with troublesome symptoms when recumbent • Avoid late meals • Avoid specific foods that precipitate symptoms	• Non-prescription antacids, H2RAs or PPIs for mild, infrequent heartburn or regurgitation. Patients should seek medical attention if symptoms persist over 2 weeks.[b] • PPIs are the preferred acid suppression therapy for GERD; H2RAs are better than placebo but not as effective as PPIs.[a] • Continuous acid suppression will be needed for most patients with GERD to both control symptoms and prevent complications.[b]

Sources: [a]Kahrilas PJ, Shaheen NJ, Vaezi MF, et al. American Gastroenterological Association Medical Position Statement on the management of gastroesophageal reflux disease. *Gastroenterology*. 2008;135:1383–1391.

[b]DeVault KR, Castell DO. Updated guidelines for the diagnosis and treatment of gastroesophageal reflux disease. *Am J Gastroenterol*. 2005;100:190–200.

FIGURE 5.2.2 Evaluation and Management of PUD

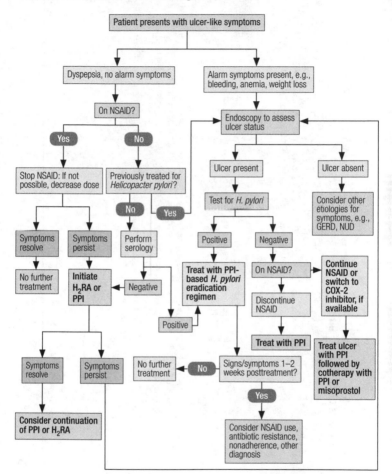

Reproduced with permission from Berardi RR, Fugit RV. Peptic ulcer disease. In: DiPiro JT, Talbert RL, Matzke GR, Posey LM, Wells BG, Yee GC, eds. *Pharmacotherapy: A Pathophysiologic Approach*. 8th ed. New York, NY: McGraw-Hill; 2011:chap 40. Figure 40-5.

TABLE 5.2.3 Acid Suppression Agents for GERD and PUD

Drug	Dosing	Comments
Proton Pump Inhibitors		
Esomeprazole (Nexium)	20–40 mg QD	• PPIs reduce recurrent ulcer risk in NSAID- treated patients by 4–6% (*Ann Int Med.* 2010; 152:101)
Dexlansoprazole (Dexilant)	30–60 mg QD	• PPI therapy is associated with increased risk of fractures (*Arch Int Med.* 2010;170:765); risk appears both dose and duration related
Lansoprazole (Prevacid, generics)	15–30 mg QD	
Pantoprazole (Protonix, generics)	40 mg QD	• Hypomagnesemia occurs with long-term therapy, measures serum [Mg^{++}] and considers Mg^{++} supplementation, especially in patients taking thiazide diuretics or digoxin
Omeprazole (Prilosec, generics)	20–40 mg QD	• PPI use associated with increased incidence of pneumonia and *Clostridium difficile* infection
Omeprazole sodium bicarbonate (Zegerid)	20–40 mg QD	
Rabeprazole (Aciphex)	20 mg QD	
H2-Receptor Antagonists		
Cimetidine (Tagamet, generics)	200–400 mg BID 800 mg QHS	• Low doses (available nonprescription) effective for episodic dyspepsia but not for GERD with esophagitis or PUD
Famotidine (Pepcid, generics)	10–20 mg BID 40 mg QHS	• Higher doses effective for mild-to-moderate GERD but less effective than PPIs for severe GERD • Multiple drug interactions with cimetidine
Nizatidine (Axid, generics)	75–150 mg BID 300 mg QHS	
Ranitidine (Zantac, generics)	75–150 mg BID 300 mg QHS	

TABLE 5.2.4 Eradication Regimens for *Helicobacter pylori*

Category	Triple Therapy	Quadruple Therapy	Sequential Therapy	Indications for *H. pylori* Testing
Acid suppression	PPI	PPI or H2RA	PPI	Clear indications: • PUD (active or documented history) • Gastric MALT lymphoma • Uninvestigated dyspepsia if age < 55 yo and no alarm symptoms[a]
Antibiotic 1	Clarithromycin 500 mg BID	Tetracycline 500 mg QID	Amoxicillin 1,000 mg BID for first 5 days	
Antibiotic 2	Amoxicillin 1,000 mg BID OR metronidazole 500 mg BID (if penicillin allergy)	Metronidazole 250–500 mg QID	Clarithromycin 250–500 mg BID PLUS metronidazole 250–500 mg BID on days 6–10	Less-established indications: • Dyspepsia without ulcer • GERD • NSAID use • Unexplained iron deficiency anemia • High risk of gastric cancer
Additional agent	—	Bismuth subsalicylate 525 mg QID	—	
Duration	10–14 days	10–14 days	10 days	
Comments	• Consider only if local *Helicobacter pylori* clarithromycin susceptibility rates are preserved • Efficacy better if BID PPI dosing used (except esomeprazole); all PPIs equally effective	• Consider first line in areas where *H. pylori* clarithromycin resistance is prevalent • May use as salvage regimen in patients who fail triple therapy • Do not substitute doxycycline for tetracycline	• High cure rates in Europe but not widely recommended first line in North America due to lack of efficacy data in that population	

Sources: (1) Chey WD, Wong BC. American College of Gastroenterology guideline on the management of Helicobacter pylori infection. *Am J Gastroenterol.* 2007;102:1808–1825. (2) PL Detail-Document, H. Pylori Treatment: An Update. Pharmacist's Letter/Prescriber's Letter. February 2012.

[a]Alarm symptoms include bleeding, anemia, early satiety, unexplained weight loss, progressive dysphagia, odynophagia, recurrent vomiting, family history of GI cancer, and previous esophagogastric malignancy.

TABLE 5.3.1 Pharmacotherapy for Complications of Cirrhosis

Clinical Situation	Pharmacotherapy	Comments
Ascites	Spironolactone 100–400 mg QD Furosemide 40–100 mg QD Albumin 25% 8 g/L of fluid removed via paracentesis	• Spironolactone directly targets hyperaldosteronism; one of the primary causes of ascites formation • Furosemide used for additional fluid removal; preferentially decreases vascular/peripheral fluid vs. peritoneal fluid; use caution with intravascular volume depletion • Ratio of 100:40 mg spironolactone: furosemide helps maintain potassium balance • Only give albumin, if ≥5 L fluid removed via paracentesis
Hepatic encephalopathy (HE)	Lactulose 15–45 mL TID up to Q 1–2 h Rifaximin 400 mg TID; max 1,200 mg/day	• Titrate lactulose to 3–4 soft bowel movements/day or as tolerated by patient • Ammonia levels do not correlate with level of impairment; assess patient symptoms • Consider rifaximin in those refractory to or intolerant of lactulose
Hepatorenal syndrome (HRS)	Albumin 25% 1 g/kg day 1; then 20–40 g/day Midodrine 5–7.5 mg TID up to 12.5 mg TID Octreotide 100 µg SQ TID up to 200 µg TID	• Discontinue if serum albumin ≥4.5 g/L
Portal hypertension	Propranolol 10 mg BID up to 80 mg/day Nadolol 20 mg QD up to 160 mg QD	• Decrease risk of variceal bleeding secondary to portal hypertension • Goal: Decrease HR by 25% or to 55–60 BPM (noninvasive surrogate marker for portal hypertension) • Initiate at low doses and titrate slowly; cirrhotic patients often have low BP at baseline
Spontaneous bacterial peritonitis (SBP)	Cefotaxime 2 g IV Q 8 h Ceftriaxone 1 g IV Q 12 h or 2 g Q 24 h Piperacillin/tazobactam 3.375 g IV Q6 h Albumin 25% 1.5 g/kg on day 1; 1 g/kg day 3	• Primarily *Escherichia coli*, *Klebsiella pneumoniae*, *Streptococcus pneumoniae*—monomicrobial; narrow antibiotic spectrum when pathogen identified • Alternative prophylactic ceftriaxone dose during variceal bleeding is 1 g IV QD • Albumin decreases incidence of HRS in patients with SBP
Long-term SBP prophylaxis	Ciprofloxacin 750 mg Q week Trimethoprim/sulfamethoxazole 1 DS tab 5X/ week	• Decreases mortality in those with prior episode of SBP • Daily vs. intermittent therapy may be preferred due to resistance concerns
Variceal bleeding	Octreotide 50–100 µg IV bolus, then 25–50 mg/h continuous infusion Prophylactic antibiotics: see empiric therapy for SBP above	• Duration controversial; continue at least 24 h after banding of varices; some recommend 5 days total • Prophylactic antibiotics recommended during acute variceal bleeding with or without ascites

SECTION

6

Pulmonology

ABBREVIATIONS

CAT	COPD assessment test	MDI	Metered-dose inhaler
DPI	Dry powder inhaler	mMRC	Modified British Medical Research Council questionnaire
FEV1	Forced expiratory flow in 1 second		
FVC	Forced vital capacity	NAEPP	National Asthma Education and Prevention Program
GOLD	Global initiative for chronic obstructive lung disease		
		PEF	Peak expiratory flow
ICS	Inhaled corticosteroid	PDE-4	Phosphodiesterase 4
ICU	Intensive care unit	SABA	Short-acting beta agonist
LABA	Long-acting beta agonist	SAMA	Short-acting muscarinic antagonist
LAMA	Long-acting muscarinic antagonist	SaO_2	Arterial oxygen saturation
LTRA	Leukotriene receptor antagonist		

FIGURE 6.1.1 Hospital Management of Acute Asthma Exacerbations

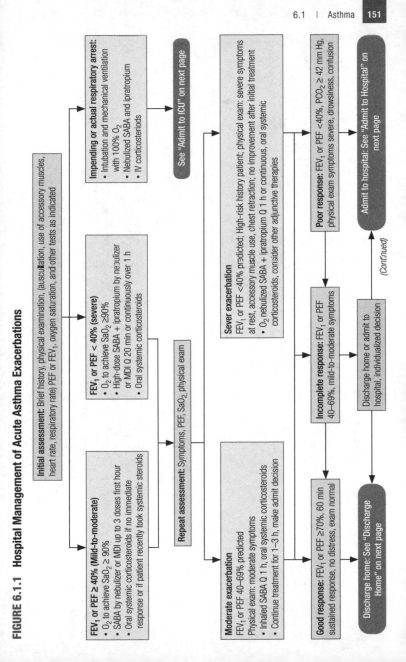

Initial assessment: Brief history, physical examination, (auscultation, use of accessory muscles, heart rate, respiratory rate) PEF or FEV₁, oxygen saturation, and other tests as indicated

FEV₁ or PEF ≥ 40% (Mild-to-moderate)
- O₂ to achieve SaO₂ ≥ 90%
- SABA by nebulizer or MDI up to 3 doses first hour
- Oral systemic corticosteroids if no immediate response or if patient recently took systemic steroids

FEV₁ or PEF < 40% (severe)
- O₂ to achieve SaO₂ ≥90%
- High-dose SABA + ipratropium by nebulizer or MDI Q 20 min or continuously over 1 h
- Oral systemic corticosteroids

Impending or actual respiratory arrest:
- Intubation and mechanical ventilation with 100% O₂
- Nebulized SABA and ipratropium
- IV corticosteroids

See "Admit to ICU" on next page

Repeat assessment: Symptoms, PEF, SaO₂, physical exam

Moderate exacerbation
FEV₁ or PEF 40–69% predicted
Physical exam: moderate symptoms
- Inhaled SABA Q 1 h, oral systemic corticosteroids
- Continue treatment for 1–3 h, make admit decision

Sever exacerbation
FEV₁ or PEF <40% predicted; High-risk history patient; physical exam: severe symptoms at rest, accessory muscle use, chest retraction; no improvement after initial treatment
- O₂ nebulized SABA + ipratropium Q 1 h or continuous, oral systemic corticosteroids, consider other adjunctive therapies

Good response: FEV₁ or PEF ≥70%, 60 min sustained response, no distress, exam normal

Incomplete response: FEV₁ or PEF 40–69%, mild-to-moderate symptoms

Poor response: FEV₁ or PEF <40%, PCO₂ ≥ 42 mm Hg, physical exam symptoms severe, drowsiness, confusion

Discharge home or admit to hospital, individualized decision

Admit to hospital: See "Admit to Hospital" on next page

Discharge home: See "Discharge Home" on next page

(Continued)

FIGURE 6.1.1 Hospital Management of Acute Asthma Exacerbations *(Continued)*

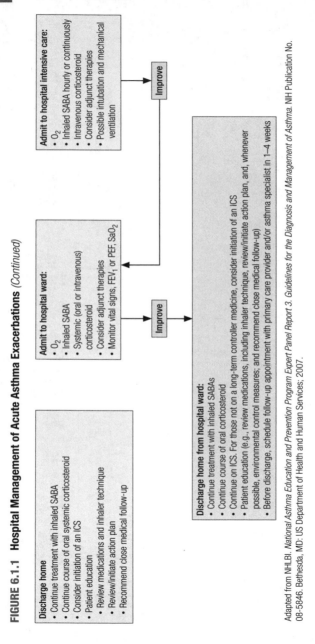

Discharge home
- Continue treatment with inhaled SABA
- Continue course of oral systemic corticosteroid
- Consider initiation of an ICS
- Patient education
- Review medications and inhaler technique
- Review/initiate action plan
- Recommend close medical follow-up

Admit to hospital ward:
- O_2
- Inhaled SABA
- Systemic (oral or intravenous) corticosteroid
- Consider adjunct therapies
- Monitor vital signs, FEV_1 or PEF, SaO_2

Admit to hospital intensive care:
- O_2
- Inhaled SABA hourly or continuously
- Intravenous corticosteroid
- Consider adjunct therapies
- Possible intubation and mechanical ventilation

Improve

Improve

Discharge home from hospital ward:
- Continue treatment with inhaled SABAs
- Continue course of oral corticosteroid
- Continue on ICS. For those not on a long-term controller medicine, consider initiation of an ICS
- Patient education (e.g., review medications, including inhaler technique, review/initiate action plan, and, whenever possible, environmental control measures; and recommend close medical follow-up)
- Before discharge, schedule follow-up appointment with primary care provider and/or asthma specialist in 1–4 weeks

Adapted from NHLBI. *National Asthma Education and Prevention Program Expert Panel Report 3. Guidelines for the Diagnosis and Management of Asthma.* NIH Publication No. 08-5846. Bethesda, MD: US Department of Health and Human Services; 2007.

TABLE 6.1.2 Drug Dosing in Acute Asthma Exacerbations

Medications	Adult Dose	Children Dose (≤12 Years Old)	Comments
SABAs			
Albuterol nebulizer solution	2.5–5 mg every 20 min for 3 doses, then 2.5–10 mg every 1–4 h PRN, or 10–15 mg/h continuously	0.15 mg/kg (minimum dose 2.5 mg) every 20 min for 3 doses, then 0.15–0.3 mg/kg (up to 10 mg) every 1–4 h PRN, or 0.5 mg/kg/h by continuous nebulization	Directly supervised MDI is equivalent to nebulizer for most patients, no data in most severe patients however (*Chest.* 2005;127:335)
Albuterol MDI	4–8 puffs every 30 min up to 4 h, then every 1–4 h PRN	4–8 puffs every 20 min for 3 doses, then every 1–4 h PRN	Use valved holding chamber-type spacer for children ≤4 years old.
Levalbuterol (Xopenex) nebulizer solution	1.25–2.5 mg every 20 min for 3 doses, then 2.5–5 mg every 1–4 h PRN, or 5–7.5 mg/h continuously	0.075 mg/kg (minimum dose 1.25 mg) every 20 min for 3 doses, then 0.075–0.15 mg/kg (up to 5 mg) every 1–4 h PRN, or 0.25 mg/kg/h by continuous nebulization	Majority of studies indicate no efficacy or tolerability advantage vs. albuterol (*Formulary.* 2009;44:108); individual exceptions may be encountered; 2.5 mg albuterol = 1.25 mg levalbuterol
Levalbuterol MDI (Xopenex)	4–8 puffs every 30 min up to 4 h, then every 1–4 h PRN	4–8 puffs every 20 min for 3 doses, then every 1–4 h PRN	
Short-Acting Anticholinergics (SAMAs)			
Ipratropium bromide nebulizer solution	500 µg every 30 min for 3 doses, then every 2–4 h PRN	250 µg every 20 min for 3 doses, then 250 µg every 2–4 h	Must use with albuterol. May mix in same nebulizer with 0.5 mL albuterol 0.5% solution.
Ipratropium bromide MDI (Atrovent)	4–8 puffs PRN every 2–4 h	4–8 puffs every 20 min for 3 doses, then every 2–4 h	Use valved holding chamber-type spacer for children ≤4 years old.
Corticosteroids			
Prednisone tablets/ Prednisolone oral solution (15 mg/5 mL)	40–80 mg/day PO in 1–2 doses	1–2 mg/kg (up to 60 mg/day) PO in 2 divided doses	Give until PEF is 70% predicted/personal best; 7–10-day courses do not need to be tapered in most patients, especially if they are taking an ICS
Methylprednisolone	32–64 mg/day PO in 1–2 doses 40–80 mg/day IV in 1–2 doses	2–4 mg/kg (up to 60 mg/day) IV	Reserve IV for NPO or severe exacerbation requiring ICU management and/or intubation. Depo-Medrol 160 mg IM at discharge equivalent to 8 days PO taper (*Chest.* 2004;126:362)

TABLE 6.1.3 Classification of Asthma Severity in Patients Not Taking Long-Term Control Medications

Children 0–11 Years of Age

	Components	Intermittent	Mild Persistent	Moderate Persistent	Severe Persistent
Impairment	Symptom frequency	≤2 days/week	>2 days/week but not daily	Daily	Throughout the day
	Nighttime awakenings (0–4 years)	None	Once or twice per month	3–4 times per month	>Once per week
	Nighttime awakenings (5–11 years)	≤twice per month	3–4 times per month	>Once per week but not nightly	Often 7 times per week
	SABA use for symptoms	≤2 days/week	>2 days/week but not daily	Daily	Several times per day
	Interference with normal activity	None	Minor limitation	Some limitation	Extremely limited
	Lung function (5–11 years)	FEV₁ >80% FEV₁/FVC >85%	FEV₁ >80% FEV₁/FVC >80%	FEV₁ 60%–80% FEV₁/FVC 75%–80%	FEV₁ <60% FEV₁/FVC <75%
Risk	Exacerbation frequency (0–4 years)	0–1 per year	≥2 in 6 months or ≥4 wheezing episodes per year lasting >1 day		
	Exacerbation frequency (5–11 years)	0–2 per year	>2 in 1 year		
	Step for initiating treatment	Step 1	Step 2	Step 3 and consider short course of systemic oral corticosteroids	

Adults and Youth ≥12 Years Old					
Components		Intermittent	Mild Persistent	Moderate Persistent	Severe Persistent
Impairment	Symptom frequency	≤2 days/week	>2 days/week but not daily	Daily	Throughout the day
	Nighttime awakenings (0–4 years)	≤2 times/month	3–4 times per month	> Once per week but not nightly	Often 7 times per week
	SABA use for symptoms	≤2 days/week	>2 days/week but not >once per day	Daily	Several times per day
	Interference with normal activity	None	Minor limitation	Some limitation	Extremely limited
	Lung function	FEV_1 >80% FEV_1/FVC normal	FEV_1 >80% FEV_1/FVC normal	FEV_1 60–80% FEV_1/FVC reduced 5%	FEV_1 <60% FEV_1/FVC reduced >5%
Risk	Exacerbation frequency	0–2 per year	>2 in 1 year		
	Step for initiating treatment	Step 1	Step 2	Step 3 and consider short course of systemic oral corticosteroids	Step 4 or 5

Adapted from NHLBI. *National Asthma Education and Prevention Program, Expert Panel Report 3. Guidelines for the Diagnosis and Management of Asthma.* NIH Publication No. 08-5846. Bethesda, MD: US Department of Health and Human Services; 2007:72–77.

TABLE 6.1.4 Recommendations for Chronic Asthma Pharmacotherapy in Children and Adults

Step	Age 0–4 Years Preferred	Age 0–4 Years Alternative	Age 5–11 Years Preferred	Age 5–11 Years Alternative	Adults and Youth Age ≥12 Years Preferred	Adults and Youth Age ≥12 Years Alternative
1	SABA PRN	N/A	SABA PRN	N/A	SABA PRN	N/A
2	Low-dose ICS	Montelukast or cromolyn	Low-dose ICS	LTRA, cromolyn, or theophylline	Low-dose ICS	LTRA, cromolyn, or theophylline
3	Medium-dose ICS	N/A	Medium-dose ICS	Low-dose ICS + either LABA, LTRA, or theophylline	Medium-dose ICS or low-dose ICS + LABA	Low-dose ICS + either LABA, LTRA, theophylline, or zileuton
4	Medium-dose ICS + either montelukast or LABA	N/A	Medium-dose ICS + LABA	Medium-dose ICS + either LTRA or theophylline	Medium-dose ICS + LABA	Medium-dose ICS + either LABA, LTRA, theophylline, or zileuton
5	High-dose ICS + either montelukast or LABA	N/A	High-dose ICS + LABA	High-dose ICS + either LTRA or theophylline	High-dose ICS + LABA and consider omalizumab in patients with allergic asthma	N/A
6	High-dose ICS + either montelukast or LABA + oral corticosteroids	N/A	High-dose ICS + LABA + oral corticosteroid	High-dose ICS + either LTRA or theophylline + oral corticosteroid	High-dose ICS + LABA + oral corticosteroid, and consider omalizumab in patients with allergic asthma	N/A

Other Measures						
SABA PRN		Use for short-term symptom relief in all patients. May give Q 20 min × 3 in acute situations.				
SQ allergy immunotherapy		Consider in all patients >4 years old with allergy triggers at treatment step 2 or above.				

Asses Control						
Step up treatment		If inadequate control by symptoms or if using SABA >2 times per week. Assess compliance with therapy and environmental measures.				
Step down treatment		If well controlled for 3 months.				

Adapted from NHLBI. *National Asthma Education and Prevention Program, Expert Panel Report 3. Guidelines for the Diagnosis and Management of Asthma. NIH Publication No. 08-5846.* Bethesda, MD: US Department of Health and Human Services; 2007:305, 306, and 343.

TABLE 6.1.5 Drug Products and Dosing in Chronic Asthma Management

Medications	Products	Adult Dose	Children Dose (≤12 Years Old)	Comments
SABAs				
Albuterol nebulizer solution	0.021% (0.63 mg/3 mL); 0.042% (1.25 mg/3 mL); 0.083% (2.5 mg/3 mL); 0.5% (2.5 mg/0.5 mL)	2.5–5 mg Q 4–6 h PRN	0.63–1.25 mg Q 4–6 h PRN	
Albuterol MDI	Ventolin HFA, Proventil HFA, ProAir HFA (all are 90 μg/puff)	2 puffs Q 4–6 h PRN	1–2 puffs Q 4–6 h PRN	Use valved holding chamber-type spacer for children ≤4 years old
Levalbuterol nebulizer solution	Xopenex 0.31 mg/3 mL; 0.63 mg/3 mL; 1.25 mg/3 mL; 1.25 mg/0.5 mL	1.25–2.5 mg Q 6–8 h PRN	0.31–0.63 mg Q 6–8 h PRN	Majority of studies indicate no efficacy or tolerability advantage vs. albuterol (*Formulary*. 2009;44:108); individual exceptions may be encountered; 2.5 mg albuterol = 1.25 mg levalbuterol
Levalbuterol MDI	Xopenex HFA (45 μg/puff)	2 puffs Q 4–6 h PRN	1–2 puffs Q 4–6 h PRN	
Pirbuterol MDI	Maxair Autohaler	2 puffs Q 4–6 h PRN	Not recommended	
Long-Acting β₂-Agonists (LABAs)				
Formoterol DPI	Foradil Aerolizer 12 μg/capsule	1 capsule inhaled via Aerolizer device Q 12 h	1 capsule inhaled via Aerolizer device Q 12 h	LABAs not recommended without ICS due to increased asthma related mortality
Salmeterol DPI	Serevent Diskus 50 μg/inhalation	1 inhalation Q 12 h	1 inhalation Q 12 h	
Mast Cell Stabilizer				
Cromolyn sodium nebulizer solution	20 mg/2 mL	20 mg 3–4 times per day	20 mg 3–4 times per day	Use 2–4 weeks to be effective. Loses efficacy with long-term use
Short-Acting Anticholinergics (SAMAs)				
Ipratropium nebulizer solution	0.03% (0.5 mg/2.5 mL)	0.5 mg Q 6–8 h PRN	0.25–0.5 mg Q 6–8 h PRN	Not as effective as SABAs in chronic asthma; only use as a replacement for patients who cannot tolerate SABAs or in addition to an SABA in acute asthma
Ipratropium MDI	Atrovent HFA 17 μg/inhalation	2 inhalations Q 6 h PRN	1–2 inhalations Q 6 h PRN	

(Continued)

TABLE 6.1.5   Drug Products and Dosing in Chronic Asthma Management *(Continued)*

Medications	Products	Adult Dose	Children Dose (≤12 Years Old)	Comments
Leukotriene Modifiers (LTRAs)				
Montelukast	Singulair 10 mg tablet, 4 mg chewable, 5 mg chewable, 4 mg granules	10 mg QD	6 months–5 years: 4 mg QPM 5–12 years: 5 mg QPM	
Zafirlukast	Accolate 10 mg tablet, 20 mg tablet	20 mg BID	5–12 years: 10 mg BID	
Zileuton	Zyflo CR 1200 mg tablet	1200 mg BID	Not recommended	AST/ALT >3 times normal occurs in 3% of patients; monitor LFTs monthly for the first 3 months of therapy
IgE inhibitor				
Omalizumab	Xolair 150 mg injection	See Table 6.1.9	Not recommended	
LABA/ICS Combination Products (see Table 6.1.6 for ICS only products)				
Salmeterol/ fluticasone DPI	Advair Diskus 100/50, 250/50 and 500/50 (fluticasone µg/salmeterol µg)	1 inhalation Q 12 h	1 inhalation Q 12 h (100/50 max if 4–11 years old)	
Salmeterol/ fluticasone MDI	Advair HFA 45/21, 115/21 and 230/21 (fluticasone µg/salmeterol µg)	2 puffs Q 12 h	2 puffs Q 12 h	
Formoterol/ budesonide MDI	Symbicort 80/4.5 or 160/4.5 (budesonide µg/ formoterol µg)	2 inhalations Q 12 h	2 inhalations Q 12 h (max dose 80/4.5, not for use <5 years old)	Patients on low-to-medium-dose ICS should take the 80/4.5 µg dose; patients on medium to high-dose ICS should take the 160/4.5 µg (Prod Info: *Symbicort*, 2010)
Methylxanthines				
Theophylline	Theo-24 extended release capsules (Q 24 h) 100, 200, 300, and 400 mg; Uniphyl controlled release tablets (Q 24 h) 400 and 600 mg; Elixophyllin elixir 80 mg/15 mL; (generics) extended release tablets (Q 12 h) 100, 200, 300, 400, 450, and 600 mg.	See Figure 6.1.7 for dosing initiation, titration and monitoring	See Figure 6.1.7 for dosing initiation, titration and monitoring	Theophylline is a narrow therapeutic index drug and should be considered as additive therapy for patients not controlled on the preferred agents. Common adverse effects include nausea, insomnia, tremors, and anxiety. For clinically important drug interactions see Table 6.1.8

TABLE 6.1.6 Inhaled Corticosteroid Comparative Dosing[a]

Medication	Products	Low Dose	Medium Dose	High Dose
Children 0–4 Years of Age				
Budesonide suspension[b]	Pulmicort Respules 0.25 mg/2 mL (2 mL); 0.5 mg/2 mL (2 mL); 1 mg/2 mL (2 mL)	0.25–0.5 mg QD (or split BID)	0.75–1 mg QD (or split BID)	>1 mg QD
Fluticasone MDI	Flovent HFA 44, 110, or 220 µg/inhalation	88 µg BID[c]	110–176 µg BID	>176 µg BID
Children 5–11 Years of Age				
Beclomethasone MDI	QVAR 40 or 80 µg/inhalation	40–80 µg BID	120–160 µg BID	>160 µg BID
Budesonide DPI	Pulmicort Flexhaler 90 or 180 µg/inhalation	90–180 µg BID	270–360 µg BID	>360 µg BID
Budesonide suspension[b]	Pulmicort Respules 0.25 mg/2 mL (2 mL); 0.5 mg/2 mL (2 mL); 1 mg/2 mL (2 mL)	0.5 mg QD (or split BID)	1 mg QD (or split BID)	2 mg QD (or split BID)
Ciclesonide MDI	Alvesco 80 or 160 µg/inhalation	80 µg QD-BID	160 µg BID	>160 µg BID
Flunisolide MDI	Aerospan 80 µg/inhalation	80 µg BID	160 µg BID	>160 µg BID
Fluticasone MDI	Flovent HFA 44, 110 or 220 µg/inhalation	44–88 µg BID[c]	110–176 µg BID	>176 µg BID

(Continued)

TABLE 6.1.6 Inhaled Corticosteroid Comparative Dosing *(Continued)*

Medication	Products	Low Dose	Medium Dose	High Dose
Adults and Youth ≥12 years of Age				
Beclomethasone MDI	QVAR 40 or 80 μg/inhalation	40–160 μg BID	200–240 μg BID	> 240 μg BID
Budesonide DPI	Pulmicort Flexhaler 90 or 180 μg/inhalation	90–270 μg BID	360–540 μg BID	>540 μg BID
Ciclesonide MDI	Alvesco 80 or 160 μg/inhalation	80 μg QD-BID	160 μg BID	>160 μg BID
Flunisolide MDI	Aerospan 80 μg/inhalation	160 μg BID	240–320 μg BID	>320 μg BID
Fluticasone MDI	Flovent HFA 44, 110 or 220 μg/inhalation	44–132 μg BID	176–220 μg BID	>220 μg BID
Mometasone DPI	Asmanex Twisthaler 110 or 220 μg/inhalation	220 μg QD	440 μg QD	>440 μg QD

Sources: (1) NHLBI, Expert Panel Report 3. Guidelines for the Diagnosis and Management of Asthma. NIH Publication No. 08-5846. (2) *Global Strategy for Asthma Management and Prevention,* Global Initiative for Asthma (GINA) 2011. http://www.ginasthma.org/. (3) Inhaled corticosteroid dose comparison. Pharmacist's Letter/Prescriber's Letter 2009;25(8):250801.

[a]ICS Pearls: Initial symptom improvement takes 1–2 weeks with peak improvement in 4–6 weeks. Improvement in FEV1 and PEF can be seen in 3–6 weeks. Bronchial hyperresponsiveness will improve after 2–3 weeks with peak improvement in 1–3 months. Exercise challenge sensitivity improves after 4 weeks. In well controlled patients with mild asthma, taking an inhaled ICS as needed for symptom control along with albuterol may provide similar control as scheduled ICS with less overall steroid exposure (*JAMA* 2012;308:987, *Lancet* 2011;377:650)

[c]May mix with albuterol (0.5% solution), levalbuterol (1.25 mg/5 mL), or ipratropium in the same nebulizer. Use only with jet nebulizers.

[d]Use higher dose of fluticasone HFA (88 μg BID) with face mask valved chamber-type spacer due to reduced drug delivery.

**FIGURE 6.1.7 Oral Sustained-Release Theophylline Dose Titration in Adults and Children >1 Year Old Without Factors Effecting Theophylline Clearance*[a]*

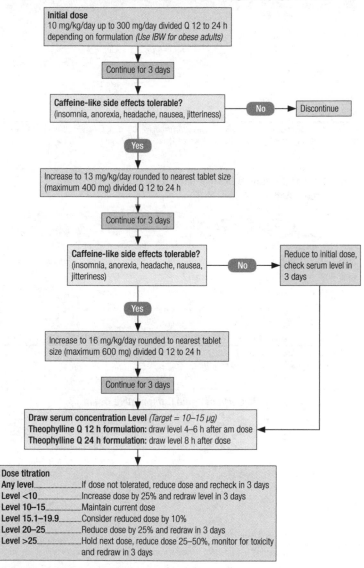

*[a]See table 6.1.8 for factors effecting theophylline clearance.

TABLE 6.1.8 Factors Altering Theophylline Clearance

Decreased Clearance	Decrease (%)	Increased Clearance	Increase (%)
Cimetidine	−25 to −60	Rifampin	+53
Erythromycin, clarithromycin	−25 to −50	Carbamazepine	+50
Allopurinol	−20	Phenobarbital	+34
Propranolol	−30	Phenytoin	+70
Ciprofloxacin	−20 to −50	Charcoal-broiled meat	+30
Interferon	−50	High-protein diet	+25
Thiabendazole	−65	Smoking	+40

Reproduced with permission from Kelly W, Sorkness CA. Asthma. In Dipiro JT, Talbert RL, Yee GC, et al., eds. *Pharmacotherapy: A Pathophysiologic Approach.* 8th ed. New York, NY: McGraw-Hill; 2011.

TABLE 6.1.9 Omalizumab Dosing in Adults and Youth ≥12 Years Old in Chronic Asthma

Pretreatment	30–60 kg	>60–70 kg	>70–90 kg	>90–150 kg
Serum IgE Level				
≥30–100	150 mg Q 4 weeks	150 mg Q 4 weeks	150 mg Q 4 weeks	300 mg Q 4 weeks
>100–200	300 mg Q 4 weeks	300 mg Q 4 weeks	300 mg Q 4 weeks	225 mg Q 2 weeks
>200–300	300 mg Q 4 weeks	225 mg Q 2 weeks	225 mg Q 2 weeks	300 mg Q 2 weeks
>300–400	225 mg Q 2 weeks	225 mg Q 2 weeks	300 mg Q 2 weeks	Not recommended
>400–500	300 mg Q 2 weeks	300 mg Q 2 weeks	375 mg Q 2 weeks	Not recommended
>500–600	300 mg Q 2 weeks	375 mg Q 2 week	Not recommended	Not recommended
>600–700	375 mg Q 2 week	Not recommended	Not recommended	Not recommended

Source: Product Information: XOLAIR(R) subcutaneous injection, omalizumab subcutaneous injection. Genentech, Inc, South San Francisco, CA, 2010.

TABLE 6.1.10 Systemic Corticosteroid Comparative Dosing

Steroid	Equivalent Anti-Inflammatory Dose	Relative Mineralocorticoid Activity	Duration of Biologic Activity
Hydrocortisone	20 mg	2	8–12 h
Prednisone/prednisolone	5 mg	1	12–36 h
Methylprednisolone	4 mg	0	12–36 h
Triamcinolone	4 mg	0	12–36 h
Dexamethasone	0.8 mg	0	36–54 h
Betamethasone	0.6 mg	0	36–54 h

Calculate the equipotent dose between steroids = Dose of steroid A × (equivalent dose steroid B ÷ equivalent dose steroid A)

Example: Prednisone 80 mg × (methylprednisolone 4 mg ÷ prednisone 5 mg) = methylprednisolone 64 mg.

TABLE 6.1.11   Adverse Effects of Inhaled and Systemic Corticosteroids[a]

Drug Class	Adverse Effect	Reported Incidence	Typical Onset	Comments
Systemic corticosteroids	Fragile skin/purpura	3% (in arthritis patients)	Variable	Most common in elderly. Dose and duration dependent.
	Cushingoid appearance	Common with high dose or long duration	2 months	Incidence increases with higher doses; reported in 25% of patients taking >7.5 mg prednisone daily for 6 months (*Ann Rheum Dis.* 2009;68:1119)
	Euphoria/psychosis	5%	1–2 weeks	Rare with doses <20 mg prednisone/day; typically resolves within a week of discontinuation
	Cataracts	Variable	1 year or longer	Typically develop bilaterally in posterior subcapsular area; risk is dose and duration related
	Osteoporosis	Variable	Variable	Dose and duration dependent; bone loss greatest during first 6 months. Reported fracture rate as high as 25% with long-term therapy
	Hyperglycemia	Near 100%	Immediate	
	Neutrophilia	Near 100%	4–6 h	Average CBC changes after 40 mg prednisone: WBC ↑ 4×10^3 cells/mm^3 (range 2–7 × 10^3), lymphocytes ↓70%, monocytes ↓90%, no left shift (*J Clin Invest.* 1968;47:249)
	Adrenal suppression	Dose and duration dependent	>3 weeks (if low dose)	It is unclear what dose and duration would not be expected to cause HPA suppression but risk appears low with doses <7.5–20 mg prednisone per day for <3 weeks (*J Clin Invest.* 1964;43:1824; *N Engl J Med.* 2003;348:727)
ICS	Dysphonia	~50%	1–2 weeks	Most common ICS adverse effect; minimized by mouthwashing and spitting after dose; incidence appears dose related
	Thrush	Undefined	1–2 weeks	Minimized by mouthwashing and spitting after dose and using a spacer
	Growth deceleration in children	Dose and duration dependent	Within 6 months	More common with high doses, 1–2 cm decreased growth seen in first year of therapy (*Pediatr Drugs.* 2011;13:11); final adult height was 1.2 cm shorter on average for patients receiving 400 mcg/day inhaled budesonide versus nedocromil or placebo (*N Engl J Med.* 2012;367:904.); short-term studies show less growth effect with ciclesonide vs. fluticasone (*Pediatr Allergy Immunol.* 2010;21:e199) and vs. budesonide (*Pediatr Allergy Immunol.* 2007;18:391)

[a]See Table 6.2.3 for bronchodilator adverse effects.

TABLE 6.2.1 GOLD Guideline Initial Pharmacotherapy for Stable COPD[a]

Patient Group	Spirometric Classification	Symptoms and Risk	First Choice	Second Choice	Alternative Choice[b]
A	FEV$_1$/FVC <0.70 and • GOLD 1 (FEV$_1$ >80%) or • GOLD 2 (FEV$_1$ 50–80%)	• Low risk, less symptoms • ≤1 exacerbation per year • mMRC 0–1 • CAT <10	SAMA PRN or SABA PRN	LAMA or LABA or SABA and SAMA	Theophylline
B	FEV$_1$/FVC <0.70 and • GOLD 1 (FEV$_1$ >80%) or • GOLD 2 (FEV$_1$ 50–80%)	• Low risk, more symptoms • ≤1 exacerbation per year • mMRC ≥2 • CAT ≥10	LAMA or LABA	LAMA and LABA	SABA and/or SAMA or Theophylline
C	FEV$_1$/FVC <0.70 and • GOLD 3 (FEV$_1$ 30–49%) or • GOLD 4 (FEV$_1$ <30%)	• High risk, less symptoms • ≥2 exacerbations per year • mMRC 0–1 • CAT <10	ICS and LABA or LAMA	LAMA and LABA	PDE-4 inhibitor or SABA and/or SAMA or Theophylline
D	FEV$_1$/FVC <0.70 and • GOLD 3 (FEV$_1$ 30–49%) or • GOLD 4 (FEV$_1$ <30%)	• High risk, more symptoms • ≥2 exacerbations per year • mMRC ≥2 • CAT ≥10	ICS and LABA or LAMA	ICS and LAMA or ICS and LABA and LAMA or ICS and LABA and PDE-4 inhibitor or LAMA and LABA or LAMA and PDE-4 inhibitor	Carbocysteine[c] or SABA and/or SAMA or Theophylline

Adapted by the author from the *Global Strategy for Diagnosis, Management and Prevention of COPD 2011*; used with permission from the Global Initiative for Chronic Obstructive Lung Disease (GOLD), www.goldcopd.org.

[a]Medications in each box are mentioned in alphabetical order, and therefore not necessarily in order of preference.

[b]Medications in this column can be used alone or in combination with other options in the first and second columns.

[c]Carbocysteine is not available in the United States.

TABLE 6.2.2 Drug Dosing for Stable COPD

Medication	Products	Class	Dosing	Comments
Short-Acting Bronchodilators				
Albuterol MDI (90 mg/puff)	Ventolin HFA, ProAir HFA, Proventil HFA	SABA	2 puffs Q 4–6 h PRN	SABA on an as needed basis provides similar clinical benefit to scheduled SABA with overall lower drug dose requirement (*Am J Respir Crit Care Med.* 2001;163:85)
Albuterol nebulizer solution	2.5 mg/3 mL (0.083%); 2.5 mg/0.5 mL (0.5%)	SABA	2.5 mg Q 4–6 h PRN	
Levalbuterol MDI (45 µg/puff)	Xoponex HFA	SABA	2 puffs Q 4–6 h PRN	
Levalbuterol nebulizer solution	Xoponex 1.25 mg/3 mL	SABA	1.25 mg Q 4–6 h PRN	
Pirbuterol MDI	Maxair Autohaler	SABA	2 puffs Q 4–6 h PRN	
Ipratropium (17 µg/puff)	Atrovent HFA	SAMA	2 puffs Q 6 h PRN	Ipratropium is longer acting than albuterol and both provide similar improvement in lung function; combination ipratropium/albuterol produces greater bronchodilation than either alone (*Chest.* 1994;105:1411)
Ipratropium nebulizer solution	0.25 mg/mL	SAMA	500 µg Q 6 h PRN	
Ipratropium/albuterol MDI	Combivent 0.18 mg/0.103 mg	SAMA/SABA	2 puffs Q 4–6 h PRN	
Ipratropium/albuterol nebulizer solution	0.5 mg/2.5 mL	SAMA/SABA	3 mL Q 4–6 h PRN	
Long-Acting Bronchodilators				
Arformoterol nebulizer solution	Brovana 15 µg/2 mL	LABA	15 µg BID	Neither GOLD nor NICE Guidelines favor LABA or LAMA. Modest benefits in trials vs. salmeterol in FEV₁, improvement (+0.137L vs. +0.085 L, p<0.001) after 6 months of therapy (*Chest.* 2002;122:47), time to exacerbation (145 vs. 187 days), and annual rate of exacerbation (0.64 vs. 0.72) (*N Engl J Med.* 2011;364:1093)
Formoterol DPI	Foradil Aerolizer 12 mg/capsule	LABA	1 capsule inhaled via Aerolizer device Q 12 h	
Salmeterol DPI	Serevent Diskus 50 µg/inhalation	LABA	1 inhalation Q 12 h	
Tiotropium	Spiriva Handihaler 18 µg/capsule	LAMA	1 capsule inhaled via Handihaler device BID	
Theophylline	See Table 6.1.5 for dosage forms	Methylxanthine	See Figure 6.1.7 for dosing initiation, titration, and monitoring	Theophylline is a narrow therapeutic index drug; must monitor serum levels to avoid toxicity; consider as add-on in uncontrolled patients on long-acting bronchodilator

(Continued)

TABLE 6.2.2 Drug Dosing for Stable COPD (Continued)

Medication	Products	Class	Dosing	Comments
ICS				
Budesonide DPI	Pulmicort Flexhaler 90 or 180 µg/ inhalation	ICS	360 µg BID	Majority of data in COPD is with fluticasone and budesonide. ICS efficacy without a bronchodilator is modest and limited to patients with FEV$_1$ <50% (Chest. 2010;137:318)
Fluticasone MDI	Flovent HFA 44, 110, or 220 µg/ inhalation	ICS	440 µg BID	
Mometasone DPI	Asmanex Twisthaler 110 or 220 µg/ inhalation	ICS	440 µg BID	
Fluticasone/salmeterol DPI	Advair Diskus 100/50, 250/50, and 500/50 (fluticasone µg/salmeterol µg)	ICS/LABA combination	500/50 µg 1 inhalation BID	Combination therapy with an ICS + LABA is superior to monotherapy with ICS (Cochrane Database Sys Rev. 2007), LABA (N Engl J Med. 2007;356:775), or tiotropium (Am J Respir Crit Care Med. 2008;177:19); Some advocate combining tiotropium, ICS, and LABA, but this approach has not been studied
Fluticasone/salmeterol MDI	Advair HFA 45/21, 115/21, and 230/21 (fluticasone µg/salmeterol µg)	ICS/LABA combination	230/21 µg 2 inhalations BID	
Budesonide/formoterol MDI	Symbicort 80/4.5 or 160/4.5 (budesonide µg/ formoterol µg)	ICS/LABA combination	160/4.5 µg 2 inhalations BID	
PDE-4 Inhibitor[a]				
Roflumilast	Daliresp 500 µg tablet	PDE-4 inhibitor	500 µg QD	Improves FEV$_1$ when combined with LABA or LAMA (Lancet. 2009;374:695); reduced exacerbations in patients with chronic bronchitis, but reduction not significant when patients with emphysema were included in the analysis (Br J Pharmacol. 2011;163:53)

Sources: (1) Global Strategy for the Diagnosis, Management and Prevention of COPD. Global Initiative for Chronic Obstructive Lung Disease (GOLD) 2011. http://www.goldcopd.org
(2) National Clinical Guideline Centre (2010). Chronic Obstructive Pulmonary Disease: Management of Chronic Obstructive Pulmonary Disease in Adults in Primary and Secondary Care.
London: National Clinical Guideline Centre. http://guidance.nice.org.uk/CG101/Guidance/pdf/English
[a]Recommended as second line agent in combination with LAMA or LABA in GOLD C or in the combinations noted in table 6.2.1 for GOLD D patients by the 2013 update of the GOLD COPD Guidelines (http://www.goldcopd.org)

TABLE 6.2.3 Adverse Effects of Bronchodilators[a]

Medication Class	Common	Severe or Noteworthy	Comments
SABA	Tremor (7%), tachycardia, anxiety	Hypokalemia, angina, tachyarrhythmia	Average increase is 10–15 bpm; angina and tachyarrhythmia are rare (a few case reports for each)
LABA	Headache (17%), tremor (8%)	Hypertension (2%), rash (1–3%), dizziness (2%), hyperglycemia (1%)	
Methylxanthines	Caffeine-like side effects (nausea, jitteriness, insomnia, headache, anorexia)	Toxicity-related side effects (theophylline level >20 µg/mL): vomiting, hypokalemia, hyperglycemia, seizures, tachycardia, ventricular arrhythmia	Incidence of specific theophylline side effects is poorly defined; vomiting with toxicity is typically forceful and intractable; seizures can be difficult to control in adults and are associated with significant mortality in the elderly
Ipratropium (SAMA)	Bitter taste (20%), xerostomia (4%)	Urinary retention, mydriasis (rare)	Mydriasis has been reported in several case reports and is usually associated with topical exposure from mask nebulization
Tiotropium (LAMA)	Xerostomia (16%), constipation (4%)	Rash (2%), myalgia (1%), dysphonia (1%)	Two studies raised concern about cardiovascular death with ipratropium and tiotropium; however, the FDA ruled the drugs were safe after reviewing these and other studies in 2010

[a]See Table 6.1.11 for ICS and systemic corticosteroid adverse effects.

FIGURE 6.2.4 Pharmacotherapy of COPD Exacerbations

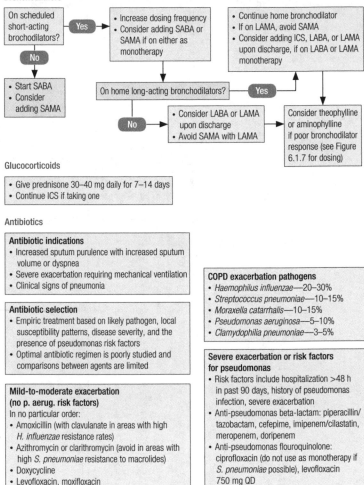

Bronchodilators

```
┌─────────────────┐       ┌──────────────────────────┐   ┌──────────────────────────────┐
│ On scheduled    │  Yes  │ • Increase dosing frequency│   │ • Continue home bronchodilator│
│ short-acting    │──────→│ • Consider adding SABA or │   │ • If on LAMA, avoid SAMA      │
│ brochodilators? │       │   SAMA if on either as    │   │ • Consider adding ICS, LABA,  │
└─────────────────┘       │   monotherapy             │   │   or LAMA upon discharge,     │
      No                  └──────────────────────────┘   │   if on LABA or LAMA          │
                                                         │   monotherapy                 │
┌─────────────────┐                                      └──────────────────────────────┘
│ • Start SABA    │       ┌──────────────────────────────────┐   Yes
│ • Consider      │       │ On home long-acting bronchodilators?│──────
│   adding SAMA   │       └──────────────────────────────────┘
└─────────────────┘                      No
                          ┌──────────────────────────┐   ┌──────────────────────────┐
                          │ • Consider LABA or LAMA  │   │ Consider theophylline    │
                          │   upon discharge         │   │ or aminophylline         │
                          │ • Avoid SAMA with LAMA   │   │ if poor bronchodilator   │
                          └──────────────────────────┘   │ response (see Figure     │
                                                         │ 6.1.7 for dosing)        │
                                                         └──────────────────────────┘
```

Glucocorticoids

- Give prednisone 30–40 mg daily for 7–14 days
- Continue ICS if taking one

Antibiotics

Antibiotic indications
- Increased sputum purulence with increased sputum volume or dyspnea
- Severe exacerbation requiring mechanical ventilation
- Clinical signs of pneumonia

Antibiotic selection
- Empiric treatment based on likely pathogen, local susceptibility patterns, disease severity, and the presence of pseudomonas risk factors
- Optimal antibiotic regimen is poorly studied and comparisons between agents are limited

Mild-to-moderate exacerbation (no p. aerug. risk factors)
In no particular order:
- Amoxicillin (with clavulanate in areas with high *H. influenzae* resistance rates)
- Azithromycin or clarithromycin (avoid in areas with high *S. pneumoniae* resistance to macrolides)
- Doxycycline
- Levofloxacin, moxifloxacin

COPD exacerbation pathogens
- *Haemophilus influenzae*—20–30%
- *Streptococcus pneumoniae*—10–15%
- *Moraxella catarrhalis*—10–15%
- *Pseudomonas aeruginosa*—5–10%
- *Clamydophilia pneumoniae*—3–5%

Severe exacerbation or risk factors for pseudomonas
- Risk factors include hospitalization >48 h in past 90 days, history of pseudomonas infection, severe exacerbation
- Anti-pseudomonas beta-lactam: piperacillin/tazobactam, cefepime, imipenem/cilastatin, meropenem, doripenem
- Anti-pseudomonas flouroquinolone: ciprofloxacin (do not use as monotherapy if *S. pneumoniae* possible), levofloxacin 750 mg QD

Sources: (1) *Global Strategy for the diagnosis Management and Prevention of COPD*, Global initiative for Chronic Obstructive Lung Disease (GOLD) 2013. http://www.goldcopdorg (2) National Clinical Guideline Centre (2010). Chronic Obstructive Pulmonary Disease Management of Chronic Obstructive Pulmonary Disease in Adults in Primary and Secondary Care. London: National Clinical Guideline Centre. http://guidancenice org.uk/CG101.Guidance/pdf/English (3) Sethi, S, Murphy, TF. Infection in the pathogenesis and course of chronic obstructive pulmonary disease. *N Engl J Med*. 2008;359:2355.

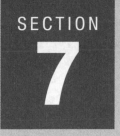

SECTION 7

Nephrology

ABBREVIATIONS			
ACEI	Angiotensin-converting enzyme inhibitor	CKD	Chronic kidney disease
		25(OH)D	25 Hydroxyvitamin D (calcidiol)
ARB	Angiotensin receptor blocker	1,25(OH)2D	1,25 Dihydroxyvitamin D (calcitriol)
BB	Beta-blocker		
CCB	Calcium channel blocker		

TABLE 7.1.1 Pharmacotherapy for Management of CKD Complications

Complication	Pharmacotherapy	Comments
Hypertension	ACEIs/ARBs first line	• Target blood pressure is <130/80 mm Hg • Most patients will require multiple agents; choose additional agents based on comorbid illnesses (see Table 1.1.2); thiazide diuretic (if CrCl > 30 mL/min) preferred second agent if no other compelling indications; CCB or BB preferred third agents (Am J Kidney Dis. 2004;43(Suppl 1):S1)
Proteinuria	ACEIs/ARBs	• Both ACEIs and ARBs reduce protein excretion by 35–40% (Am J Kidney Dis. 2004;43:S1) • An ACEI plus ARB regimen can decrease proteinuria greater than either alone but may worsen kidney disease (Lancet. 2008;372:547) • Spironolactone combined with an ACEI or ARB may reduce proteinuria greater than either alone (Clin J Am Soc Nephrol. 2006;1:256); monitor serum K⁺ closely with this combination • Titrate ACE/ARB to maximum tolerated dose see Table 1.1.1 for dosing), monitor serum K⁺ and SCr 1 week after initiation
Hyperlipidemia	Statins	• Target LDL-C <100 mg/dL (Am J Kidney Dis. 2005;45:S1–S153) • There is conflicting data on whether statins decrease CKD progression.
Anemia	Erythropoietin-stimulating agents (ESAs) and iron	• A trial of IV iron or 1–3 months of PO iron can be considered for any patient with TSAT ≤ 30% and ferritin ≤ 500 ng/mL (Kidney Int Suppl. 2012;2:279.) • Consider ESA if Hgb is between 9–10 g/dL, a maximum Hgb = 11.5 g/dL is appropriate for most patients (Kidney Int Suppl. 2012;2:279.) • See Tables 11.1–11.1.2 for dosing of ESAs and iron products

(Continued)

TABLE 7.1.1 Pharmacotherapy for Management of CKD Complications *(Continued)*

Complication	Pharmacotherapy	Comments
CKD mineral and bone disorder (CKD-MBD)	Activated vitamin D, vitamin D precursors or analogs; calcimimetic	• See 7.1.2 for indications and dosing • K/DOQI (2003) treatment goals: PTH = (35–70 pg/mL for CKD stage 3 or 70–110 pg/mL for CKD stage 4); serum phosphate 2.7–4.6 mg/dL; serum Ca^{++} in normal range; Ca-P product < 55 (*Am J Kidney Dis.* 2003;42:S1) • KDIGO (2009) treatment goals: PTH, serum Ca^{++} and phosphate in normal range for the assay measured (*Kidney Int.* 2009;76(Suppl 113):S1)
Hyperphosphatemia	Phosphate binders	
Metabolic acidosis	• $NaHCO_3$ tablets (650 mg = 7.7 mEq Na^+ and HCO_3^-) • Na^+ citrate solution (Bicitra = 1 mEq/L Na^+ and HCO_3^-) • Na^+/K^+ citrate solution (Polycitra = 1 mEq/L Na^+ and K^+ and 2 mEq/L HCO_3^-)	• Goal is to maintain serum $HCO_3 \cong 24$ mEq/L • Calculate base deficit: [0.5 L/kg × (weight [kg]) × [(normal CO_2) – (measured CO_2)] • Replace total deficit over several days to avoid volume overload • Once base deficit replaced, titrate maintenance dose to achieve serum $HCO_3 \cong 24$ mEq/L • Use of Na^+/K^+ citrate solution can lead to hyperkalemia

TABLE 7.1.2 Pharmacotherapy for Maintenance of Calcium and Phosphorus Homeostasis in Pre-dialysis Patients

Drug	Dosing	Comments
Vitamin D Precursors		
Cholecalciferol (vitamin D₃)	• Serum 25(OH)D = 16–30 ng/mL: 800–1000 IU PO daily	• Ergocalciferol may be preferred (Am J Kidney Dis. 2003;42:S1)
Ergocalciferol (vitamin D₂)	• Serum 25(OH)D = 16–30 ng/mL: 800 IU PO daily or 50,000 IU PO monthly	• Measure serum 25(OH)D after 6 months of therapy and reassess
	• Serum 25(OH)D = 5–15 ng/mL: 50,000 IU PO weekly × 4, then monthly	• Vitamin D precursors lose efficacy as CKD progresses due to a loss of renal conversion to activated vitamin D
	• Serum 25(OH)D <5 ng/mL: 50,000 IU PO weekly × 12, then monthly, alternatively 500,000 IU IM × 1	• Patients with osteomalacia should receive an active vitamin D product instead of a precursor
Activated Vitamin D and Analogs		
Calcitriol (Calcijex, Rocaltrol)	• 0.25 μg PO daily	• Consider activated vitamin D products if serum 25(OH)D levels >30 ng/mL and PTH elevated
Doxercalciferol (Hectorol)	• 1 μg PO daily, may increase by 0.5 mcg every 2 weeks (maximum 3.5 mcg) to achieve target iPTH decline	• Activated vitamin D products are contraindicated in CKD stage 3–4 if serum Ca⁺⁺ >9.5 mg/dL or serum phosphorus >4.6 mg/dL
Paricalcitol (Zemplar)	• 1 μg PO daily or 2 μg PO 3 × per week, adjust dose at 2–4 week intervals to achieve target iPTH decline	• Monitor serum Ca⁺⁺, phosphate every month × 3, then every 3 months; monitor PTH every 3 months × 2, then every 6 months
		• Dose conversion of paricalcitol to doxercalciferol is approximately 1 μg to 0.57 μg (Am J Nephrol. 2005;25:591)

(Continued)

TABLE 7.1.2 Pharmacotherapy for Maintenance of Calcium and Phosphorus Homeostasis in Pre-dialysis Patients *(Continued)*

Drug	Dosing	Comments
Calcimimetic		
Cinacalcet (Sensipar)	• 30–180 mg PO daily	• Use of cinacalcet in non-dialysis patients is controversial and carries an appreciable risk of hypocalcemia and hyperphosphatemia; weekly monitoring is warranted until stable, titrate dose upward every 2–4 weeks as needed • Consider for patients refractory to all other available treatments
Phosphate Binders		
Calcium acetate (Phos-Lo)	• 3–6 tablets (168 mg elemental Ca^{++} per tablet) 3 times daily with meals (0.5–1 gram elemental Ca^{++} per dose)	• Calcium products are preferred unless corrected serum Ca^{++} >10.2 mg/dL • Calcium acetate contains less elemental calcium (25% versus 40%) and is preferred for patients in whom calcium intake should be limited
Calcium carbonate	• 0.5–1 gram elemental Ca^{++} 3 times daily with meals	
Lanthanum carbonate (Fosrenal)	• 750–1500 mg 3 times daily with meals	
Sevelamer carbonate (Renvela)	• 800 mg 3 times daily with meals	

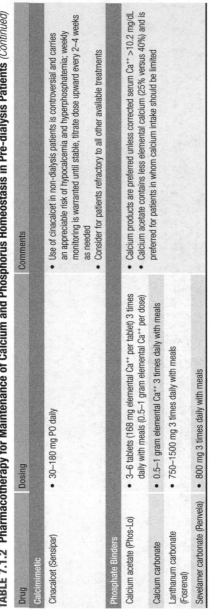

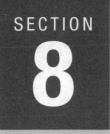

SECTION 8

Rheumatology

ABBREVIATIONS			
DMARD	Disease-modifying antirheumatic drug	MTX	Methotrexate
		NSAID	Nonsteroidal anti-inflammatory drug
HCQ	Hydroxychloroquine	TNF	Tumor necrosis factor
LEF	Leflunomide		

TABLE 8.1.1 Pharmacotherapy for Early Rheumatoid Arthritis

Prognostic Features	Treatment by Disease Activity[b]		
	Low Disease Activity	Moderate Disease Activity	High Disease Activity
No poor prognostic features[a]	DMARD monotherapy	DMARD monotherapy	DMARD monotherapy or HCQ PLUS MTX
With poor prognostic features[a]	Combination DMARD therapy: (MTX + HCQ or LEF or sulfasalazine) or (sulfasalazine + HCQ) or (MTX + HCQ + sulfasalazine)	Combination DMARD therapy: (MTX + HCQ or LEF or sulfasalazine) or (sulfasalazine − HCQ) or (MTX + HCQ + sulfasalazine)	Anti-TNF +/− MTX or combination DMARD therapy: (MTX + HCQ or LEF or sulfasalazine) or (sulfasalazine + HCQ) or (MTX + HCQ + sulfasalazine)

Source: Singh JA, Furst DE, Bharat A, et al. 2012 Update of the 2008 American College of Rheumatology Recommendations for use of disease-modifying antirheumatic drugs and biologic agents in the treatment of rheumatoid arthritis. *Arth Care Res.* 2012;64(5):625–639.

[a]Poor prognostic features: Functional limitation, extraarticular disease, bony erosions on radiograph, positive rheumatoid factor, or anticyclic citrullinated peptide antibodies.

[b]Categorized based on validated scales such as Patient Activity Scale (PAS), Clinical Disease Activity Index, or Disease Activity Score.

TABLE 8.1.2 Dosing, Adverse Effects, and Monitoring of DMARDs

Agent	Dosing	Adverse Effects	Monitoring
Nonbiologic DMARDS			
HCQ	Initial: 400–600 mg PO QD for 4–12 weeks; max 200–400 mg PO QD	• Common: GI side effects, photosensitivity, hair bleaching • Serious: Retinopathy (1% after 5–7 years of use), angioedema, hepatotoxicity, bronchospasm, exfoliative dermatitis, Stevens–Johnson syndrome, bone marrow toxicity	• Eye exam at baseline and every 5 years or sooner (some experts recommend annual exams); do not exceed the retinopathy threshold 200–400 mg QD; cumulative dose of 1,000 g is associated with retinopathy • CBC with platelet counts during prolonged therapy
MTX	10–15 mg PO once weekly, increase by 5 mg/week every 2–3 weeks to a maximum of 20–30 mg/week	• Common: Alopecia (0.5–3%), diarrhea (1–3%), nausea and vomiting (>10%), leukopenia (1–3%), thrombocytopenia (3–10%), dizziness (1–35) • Serious: Hepatic fibrosis (7%), pancytopenia (1–3%), toxic epidermal necrolysis, GI hemorrhage, stomatitis (2–10%), acquired infections	• Pregnancy category X • Hepatic function baseline and 1–2 months intervals; renal function (80–90% unchanged in urine) • Chest x-ray prior to initiation, pulmonary function testing prior to initiation
LEF (Arava)	• Loading dose: 100 mg PO QD × 3 days • Maintenance: 20 mg PO QD, reduce to 10 mg QD if not tolerated	• Common: Alopecia (9–17%), rash (10–12%), diarrhea (17–27%), mouth ulcer (3–5%), headache (7–13%) • Serious: Stevens–Johnson syndrome, toxic epidermal necrolysis, bone marrow toxicity, hepatic necrosis (increased LFTs 1.5–4.4%), opportunistic infections, interstitial lung disease	• Pregnancy category X • CBC with platelet counts and LFTs at baseline, then monthly for 6 months, then every 6–8 weeks thereafter • Signs and symptoms of interstitial lung disease and serious infection
Minocycline	100 mg PO BID	• Common: Tooth discoloration in forming teeth; dizziness (9%), vertigo, photosensitivity • Serious: Hypersensitivity, pseudotumor cerebri	• LFTs if hepatitis symptoms occur • SCr and adjustment perhaps with CKD (no guidelines)
Sulfasalazine	Initial 0.5–1 g/day PO BID Maximum dose up to 3 g QD	• Common: Pruritus (3–4%), rash (3–13%), GI complaints (up to 33%), headache (9–33%), fever (3–5%) • Serious: Stevens–Johnson syndrome (rare), bone marrow toxicity, hepatotoxicity, hypersensitivity, male infertility, interstitial pulmonary fibrosis	• CBC with platelet counts and LFTs at baseline, then every 3 months thereafter • Urinalysis for crystals

Biologic Non-TNF DMARDs

Abatacept (Orencia)	• <60 kg: 500 mg IV over 30 min, repeat doses at 2 and 4 weeks; then every 4 weeks thereafter • 60–100 kg: 750 mg IV over 30 min then similar to above • >100 kg: 1000 mg IV over 30 min then similar to above	• Common: Nausea (~10%), infections (37–54%), headache 12–18%), UTI (6%), COPD exacerbation (43%) • Serious: UTI (0.2–0.5%), pneumonia (0.2–0.5%), cancer (1.3%)	• Signs and symptoms of infection; screen for TB before starting therapy
Rituximab (Rituxan)	1000 mg IV followed by 1,000 mg IV 2 weeks later in combination with MTX repeated every 16–24 weeks	• Common: Infusion reactions, fever, lymphopenia, chills, infections • Serious: Severe infusion reactions (urticaria, hypotension, angioedema, hypoxia, bronchospasm, pulmonary infiltrates, acute respiratory distress syndrome, myocardial infarction, ventricular fibrillation, cardiogenic shock, anaphylactoid events, or death) in up to 77% with the first infusion	• Premedicate with methylprednisolone 100 mg IV 30 min prior to infusion, antihistamine and APAP • JC virus infection resulting in PML, and death can occur in rituximab-treated patients
Tocilizumab (Actemra)	• 4 mg/kg IV infusion over 1 h every 4 weeks; increase to 8 mg/kg based on clinical response (max 800 mg)	• Common: Hypertension (4–6%), rash (2–4%), diarrhea (>5%), LFT elevation (up to 48%), nasopharyngitis (4%) • Serious: Injection site reaction (5%), GI perforation, thrombocytopenia (up to 1.7%), neutropenia (up to 3.4%), anaphylaxis (0.2%), URI (6–8%), potential for malignancy	• Neutrophil count (ANC) 500–1,000/mm³, interrupt therapy and resume at 4 mg/kg when ANC is greater than 1000/mm³; increase to 8 mg/kg as clinically appropriate; absolute neutrophil count below 500/mm³, discontinue therapy • Signs and symptoms of infection, including tuberculosis, even if initial latent tuberculosis test is negative
Anakinra (Kineret)	100 mg/day SQ	• Common: Injection site reaction (71%) • Serious: Immune hypersensitivity reaction, Infectious disease (2–3%), malignant lymphoma, cardiopulmonary arrest	• Severe renal impairment or end-stage renal disease: CrCl less than 30 mL/min, 100 mg SQ every other day

(Continued)

TABLE 8.1.2 Dosing, Adverse Effects, and Monitoring of DMARDs *(Continued)*

Agent	Dosing	Adverse Effects	Monitoring
Biologic Anti-TNF DMARDs			
Adalimumab (Humira)	40 mg SQ every other week; other DMARDs may be continued during therapy; may increase to 40 mg SQ every week in patients not receiving concomitant MTX	• Common: Injection site reaction/pain (12–19%), rash (12%), antibody development, adalimumab (1–12%), antinuclear antibody positive (12%), headache (12%), sinusitis (11%), upper respiratory infection (17%) • Serious: Heart failure (<5%), aplastic anemia (rare), erythrocytosis (less than 5%), leukopenia (less than 5%), pancytopenia (less than 5%), thrombocytopenia (infrequently), immune hypersensitivity reaction (approximately 1%), risk of malignancy and infections	• Discontinue therapy if lupus-like syndrome develops • Signs/symptoms of fungal infections and other serious systemic infections during and after treatment, especially patients with a history of recurrent infection
Etanercept (Enbrel)	50 mg SQ weekly given as one 50 mg injection or two 25 mg injections in one day, or one 25 mg injection given twice weekly, 72–96 h apart	• Common: Injection site reaction (37–43%), rhinitis (12–14%), URI (17–65%) • Serious: Heart failure (0.1% or less), erythema multiforme, malignant melanoma, necrotizing fasciitis, primary cutaneous vasculitis, skin cancer, squamous cell carcinoma of skin, Stevens–Johnson syndrome, toxic epidermal necrolysis, aplastic anemia (less than 0.01%), leukopenia, neutropenia, pancytopenia (less than 0.1%), thrombocytopenia, autoimmune hepatitis (less than 1%), risk of infection and malignancy	• ESR, rheumatoid factor, and C-reactive protein may be measured for indication of efficacy • Evaluate for TB at baseline and monitor during therapy, increased risk for fungal infections, LFT during therapy, some risk for heart failure

| Certolizumab (Cimzia) | • Initial: 400 mg SQ (as 2 SQ injections of 200 mg) once and then repeat at weeks 2 and 4
• Maintenance: 200 mg SQ once every 2 weeks or 400 mg (as 2 SQ injections of 200 mg) every 4 weeks | • Common: Infections (e.g., nasopharyngitis, laryngitis, viral infection), urinary tract infections (e.g., bladder infection, bacteriuria, cystitis), and arthralgia
• Serious: Potential cardiovascular adverse effect, TB and other infections, bone marrow toxicity | • Increased risk for developing serious infections that may lead to hospitalization or death and lymphoma and other malignancies |
| Golimumab (Simponi) | 50 mg SQ once monthly in combination with MTX | • Common: Hypertension (3%), injection site reaction (6%), LFT elevation (3–4%), bronchitis (2%), sinusitis (2%), URI (16%)
• Serious: Increased risk for malignancy and infections (28% overall), optic neuritis, demyelinating disease of central nervous system, Guillain–Barré syndrome | • Baseline screening for TB
• Monitor for new or worsening heart failure |

FIGURE 8.3.1 Algorithm for Treatment of Acute Gouty Arthritis

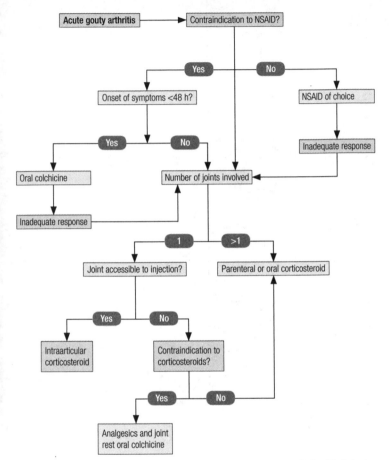

From Ernst ME, Clark EC. Chapter 102: Gout and hyperuricemia. In: DiPiro JT, Talbert RL, Yee GC, et al., eds. *Pharmacotherapy: A Pathophysiological Approach.* 8th ed. New York, NY: McGraw-Hill; 2011:1627, with permission.

TABLE 8.3.2 Pharmacotherapy for Acute and Chronic Gout

Drug	Dose	Comments
Acute Gout		
Corticosteroids	30–60 mg PO prednisone equivalent (see Table 6.1.10)	• Intraarticular injection (triamcinolone 10–40 mg or similar) preferred for single joint involvement
Colchicine	1.2 mg PO × 1, then 0.6 mg PO 1 h later	• If CrCl <30 mL/min, repeat no more than every 2 weeks • GI side effects common (nausea, vomiting, diarrhea)
NSAIDs	See Table 14.1.1	• Indomethacin historically favored NSAID though no evidence of superiority • Start early and at max doses, caution with renal insufficiency or heart failure
Chronic Gout		
Allopurinol	100–300 mg PO daily (may divide in 2–3 doses)	• Titrate up by 100 mg/day at weekly intervals to max dose (with normal renal function) of 800 mg per day to maintain uric acid level <6 mg/dL • Max 200 mg per day if CrCl 10–20 mL/min • Rash is most common side effect (1%)
Colchicine	0.6 mg PO daily	• 0.3 mg PO daily or 0.6 mg every other day if CrCl <30 mL/min
Febuxostat (Uloric)	40 mg PO daily	• Increase dose to 80 mg PO daily if uric acid level >6 mg/dL after 2 weeks • Rash most common adverse effect (0.5–1.6%)
NSAIDs	Use lowest effective dose (see Table 14.1.1)	
Probenecid	250 mg PO BID	• May titrate up to 2,000 mg per day to maintain uric acid level <6 mg/dL • Not recommended if CrCl < 50 mL/min • Avoid in patients with nephrolithiasis

FIGURE 9.1.1 Assessment and Management of Depression Algorithm

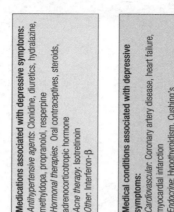

Initial assessment: At least five of the following have been present for at least 2 weeks: (1) Depressed mood, (2) markedly diminished interest or pleasure in activities, (3) significant changes in weight or appetite, (4) insomnia or hypersomnia, (5) psychomotor agitation or retardation, (6) fatigue or loss of energy, (7) feelings of worthlessness or excessive or inappropriate guilt, (8) diminished ability to think or concentrate, (9) recurrent thoughts of death or suicide. The symptoms cause clinically significant distress or impairment in daily functioning.

Medications associated with depressive symptoms:
Antihypertensive agents: Clonidine, diuretics, hydralazine, methyldopa, propranolol, resperpine
Hormonal therapies: Oral contraceptives, steroids, adrenocorticotropic hormone
Acne therapy: Isotretinoin
Other: Interferon-β

Identify comorbid conditions and medications
• Obtain a complete medical, family, and psychiatric history including previous hospitalizations and suicide
• Consider medications and medical conditions that may be contributing to symptoms
• Rule out other psychiatric disorders such as bipolar disorder. If present, refer to psychiatrist for evaluation

Medical conditions associated with depressive symptoms:
Cardiovascular: Coronary artery disease, heart failure, myocardial infarction
Endocrine: Hypothyroidism, Cushing's
Infections: HIV, mononucleosis, tuberculosis
Metabolic: Hyponatremia, hypokalemia, encephalopathy
Neurologic: Alzheimer's, epilepsy, Huntington's, multiple sclerosis, Parkinson's
Other: Anemia, systemic lupus erythematosus, malignancy

Initial treatment
• Identify target symptoms and goals of therapy
• Develop a detailed safety plan with patient in case suicidal ideation or behaviors develop
• Initiate antidepressant pharmacotherapy based on patient preference, prior response, safety, tolerability/adverse effects, comorbid disorders, potential drug interactions, pharmacokinetic parameters, and cost
• Consider administration of standardized rating scale such as QIDS-SR or PHQ-9

Weeks 1–4 assessment
Full response:
Maintain current treatment if there are no issues with tolerability
Partial or nonresponse:
1. Assess adherence
2. Increase dose if clinically indicated and if no issues with tolerability
3. For severe symptoms, consider ECT

(Continued)

FIGURE 9.1.1 Assessment and Management of Depression Algorithm *(Continued)*

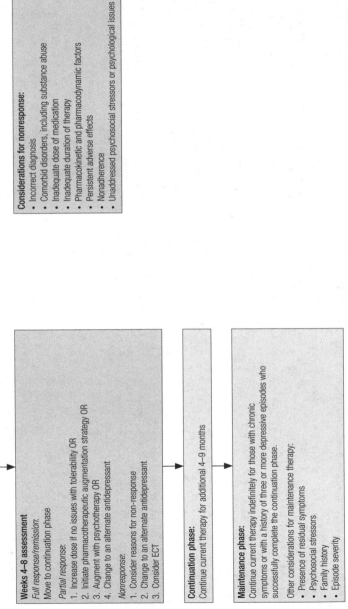

Considerations for nonresponse:
- Incorrect diagnosis
- Comorbid disorders, including substance abuse
- Inadequate dose of medication
- Inadequate duration of therapy
- Pharmacokinetic and pharmacodynamic factors
- Persistent adverse effects
- Nonadherence
- Unaddressed psychosocial stressors or psychological issues

Weeks 4–8 assessment
Full response/remission:
Move to continuation phase
Partial response:
1. Increase dose if no issues with tolerability OR
2. Initiate pharmacotherapeutic augmentation strategy OR
3. Augment with psychotherapy OR
4. Change to an alternate antidepressant
Nonresponse:
1. Consider reasons for non-response
2. Change to an alternate antidepressant
3. Consider ECT

Continuation phase:
Continue current therapy for additional 4–9 months

Maintenance phase:
Continue current therapy indefinitely for those with chronic symptoms or with a history of three or more depressive episodes who successfully complete the continuation phase.
Other considerations for maintenance therapy:
- Presence of residual symptoms
- Psychosocial stressors
- Family history
- Episode severity

Source: American Psychiatric Association. *Practice Guideline for the Treatment of Patients with Major Depressive Disorder.* 3rd ed. Arlington, VA: American Psychiatric Association; 2010.

TABLE 9.1.2 Antidepressant Drug Dosing

Medication	Dosage Forms	Usual Dosing Range	Monitoring
SSRIs			
Citalopram	Tablet, oral solution	20–40 mg/day	• Monitor ECG. Mg⁺ and K⁺ due to QTc prolongation
Escitalopram	Tablet, oral solution	10–20 mg/day	
Fluoxetine	Tablet, capsule, oral solution	20–80 mg/day	• Avoid use in elderly and those with hepatic impairment (long $t_{1/2}$)
Paroxetine	Tablet, controlled release tablet, oral suspension	10–60 mg/day	• Avoid abrupt discontinuation due to withdrawal syndrome
Sertraline	Tablet, oral solution	25–200 mg/day	
Dual Reuptake Inhibitors			
Bupropion	Immediate release tablet	300–450 mg/day, divided	• Contraindicated in seizure disorder or eating disorders
	Sustained release tablet	150–400 mg/day, divided	
	Extended release tablet	150–300 mg/day	
Duloxetine	Delayed-release capsule	20–60 mg/day	• May cause urinary hesitation • Avoid in hepatic impairment, chronic alcohol abuse or CrCl <30 mL/min
Venlafaxine	Tablet, extended release capsule, sustained release tablet	75–300 mg/day	• Monitor blood pressure • Avoid abrupt discontinuation due to withdrawal syndrome • May see a "ghost tablet" with sustained release
Desvenlafaxine	Tablet, oral disintegrating tablet	50–400 mg/day	• Avoid abrupt discontinuation due to withdrawal syndrome
TCAs			
Amitriptyline	Tablet	10–300 mg/day	• May cause blue-green urine
Desipramine	Tablet	10–300 mg/day	• May cause blue-green urine
Imipramine	Tablet, capsule	10–300 mg/day	
Nortriptyline	Capsule, oral solution	30–150 mg/day	
MAOIs			
Phenelzine	Tablet	60–90 mg/day, divided	• Required medication and dietary restrictions
Selegiline	Transdermal patch	6–12 mg/day	• Dietary restrictions for 9 and 12 mg patches
Tranylcypromine	Tablet	10–60 mg/day	• More rapid onset than tricyclics • Required medication and dietary restrictions
Isocarboxazid	Tablet	20–60 mg/day, divided	• Required medication and dietary restrictions

(Continued)

TABLE 9.1.2 Antidepressant Drug Dosing (Continued)

Medication	Dosage Forms	Usual Dosing Range	Monitoring
Novel Mechanism Agents			
Mirtazapine	Tablet, oral disintegrating tablet	15–45 mg/day	• Causes significant sedation • May increase triglycerides • Monitor weight
Nefazodone	Tablet	300–600 mg/day	• Monitor liver function, signs of hepatic failure
Trazodone	Tablet	150–600 mg/day	• Give at bedtime • Causes sedation • May cause priapism
Vilazodone	Tablet	20–40 mg/day	• Must take with food for adequate absorption

Reprinted with permission from Mascarenas CA. Major depressive disorder. In: Richardson MM, Chessman KH, Chant C, Cheng JWM, Hemstreet BA, Hume AL, et al., eds. *Pharmacotherapy Assessment Program.* 7th ed. Neurology and Psychiatry. Lenexa, KS: American College of Clinical Pharmacy;2012:7–26.

TABLE 9.1.3 Depression Augmentation Medications

Medication	Total Daily Dose (mg)	Time to Response (week)
Aripiprazole	5–15	1–4
Bupropion	300, divided	1–6
Buspirone	30–45, divided	2–6
Lithium	600–900	1–4
Mirtazapine	15–30	4
Methylphenidate	10–40	1–2
Liothyronine	0.25–0.5	1–6
Olanzapine	5–15	4–8
Risperidone	0.5–2	1–12
Quetiapine (extended release)	150–300	1–4

Reprinted with permission from Mascarenas CA. Major depressive disorder In: Richardson MM, Chessman KH, Chant C, Cheng JWM, Hemstreet BA, Hume AL, et al., eds. *Pharmacotherapy Assessment Program.* 7th ed. Neurology and Psychiatry. Lenexa, KS: American College of Clinical Pharmacy;2012, 7–26.

TABLE 9.1.4 Conditions Influencing Antidepressant Pharmacotherapy Selection

Condition	Recommended	Avoid/Caution	Comments
Benign prostatic hyperplasia		Amitriptyline Imipramine Paroxetine	Avoid due to anticholinergic effects
Eating disorders	Fluoxetine	Bupropion	Risk of seizures with bupropion
Cardiovascular disease	Sertraline	TCAs Citalopram Mirtazapine	TCAs; citalopram may cause ECG changes
Chronic pain/neuropathy	Duloxetine Venlafaxine Desvenlafaxine TCAs		
Diabetes mellitus		TCAs	May worsen glycemic control; low doses may be used in diabetic neuropathy
Dementia	Citalopram Escitalopram Sertraline	TCAs	Anticholinergic effects
Hepatic insufficiency	Desvenlafaxine	Fluoxetine Duloxetine Nefazodone	Duloxetine and nefazodone associated with hepatotoxicity
Hypertension		TCAs Venlafaxine Desvenlafaxine Duloxetine	Increased sympathetic tone
Narrow angle glaucoma		Amitriptyline Imipramine Paroxetine	Anticholinergic effects
Obesity	Bupropion SSRIs (except paroxetine) SNRIs	Mirtazapine TCAs MAOIs	
Seizures	SSRIs SNRIs	Bupropion TCAs	
Stroke	SSRIs		Caution with antiplatelets and anticoagulants
Tamoxifen	Venlafaxine Desvenlafaxine Citalopram Escitalopram	Paroxetine Fluoxetine Bupropion	CYP2D6 inhibition prevents conversion to active compound
Tobacco use	Bupropion Nortriptyline		
Underweight	Mirtazapine	Bupropion	

Reprinted with permission from Mascarenas CA. Major depressive disorder In: Richardson MM, Chessman KH, Chant C, Cheng JWM, Hemstreet BA, Hume AL, et al., eds. *Pharmacotherapy Assessment Program*. 7th ed. Neurology and Psychiatry. Lenexa, KS: American College of Clinical Pharmacy;2012:7–26.

FIGURE 9.2.1 Treatment Algorithm for Generalized Anxiety Disorder

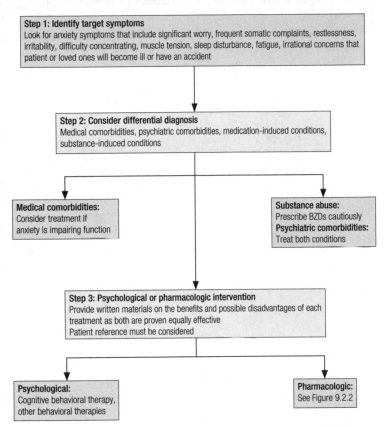

Step 1: Identify target symptoms
Look for anxiety symptoms that include significant worry, frequent somatic complaints, restlessness, irritability, difficulty concentrating, muscle tension, sleep disturbance, fatigue, irrational concerns that patient or loved ones will become ill or have an accident

Step 2: Consider differential diagnosis
Medical comorbidities, psychiatric comorbidities, medication-induced conditions, substance-induced conditions

Medical comorbidities:
Consider treatment if anxiety is impairing function

Substance abuse:
Prescribe BZDs cautiously
Psychiatric comorbidities:
Treat both conditions

Step 3: Psychological or pharmacologic intervention
Provide written materials on the benefits and possible disadvantages of each treatment as both are proven equally effective
Patient reference must be considered

Psychological:
Cognitive behavioral therapy, other behavioral therapies

Pharmacologic:
See Figure 9.2.2

Sources: Canadian Psychiatric Association clinical practice guidelines for the management of anxiety disorders. *Can J Psychiatry*. 2006;51(Suppl. 2):1S–92S; National Institute for Health and Clinical Excellence (2011) [Generalized anxiety disorder and panic disorder (with or without agoraphobia) in adults]. [113] London: National Institute for Health and Clinical Excellence.

FIGURE 9.2.2 Pharmacotherapy for Generalized Anxiety Disorder

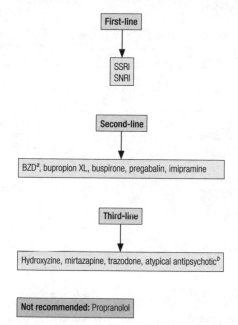

First-line

SSRI
SNRI

Second-line

BZD[a], bupropion XL, buspirone, pregabalin, imipramine

Third-line

Hydroxyzine, mirtazapine, trazodone, atypical antipsychotic[b]

Not recommended: Propranolol

Source: Canadian Psychiatric Association clinical practice guidelines for the management of anxiety disorders. *Can J Psychiatry*. 2006;51(Suppl. 2):1S–92S.

[a]BZD may be added to first-line treatments at the initiation of therapy while waiting for first-line treatment to take effect.

[b]Consider referral to mental-health specialist.

FIGURE 9.2.3 Pharmacotherapy for Generalized Anxiety Disorder Treatment Resistance

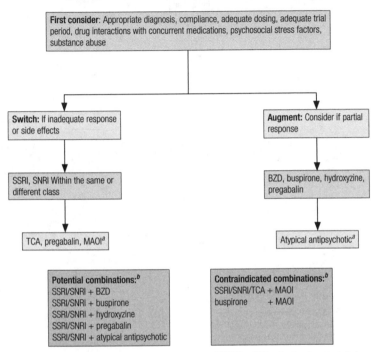

Source: World Federation of Societies of Biological Psychiatry (WFSBP) guidelines for the pharmacological treatment of anxiety, obsessive-compulsive and post-traumatic stress disorders—first revision. *World J Biol Psychiatry.* 2008;9(4):248–312.

[a]Consider referral to mental-health specialist.

[b]Canadian Psychiatric Association clinical practice guidelines for the management of anxiety disorders. *Can J Psychiatry.* 2006;51(Suppl. 2):1S–92S.

FIGURE 9.2.4 Treatment Algorithm for Panic Disorder with or without Agoraphobia

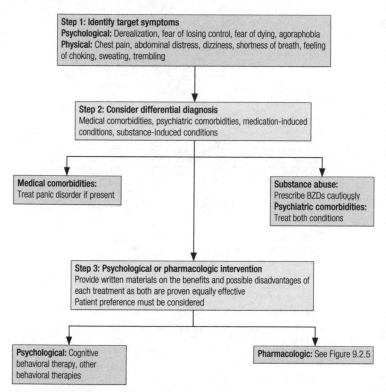

Step 1: Identify target symptoms
Psychological: Derealization, fear of losing control, fear of dying, agoraphobia
Physical: Chest pain, abdominal distress, dizziness, shortness of breath, feeling of choking, sweating, trembling

Step 2: Consider differential diagnosis
Medical comorbidities, psychiatric comorbidities, medication-induced conditions, substance-induced conditions

Medical comorbidities:
Treat panic disorder if present

Substance abuse:
Prescribe BZDs cautiously
Psychiatric comorbidities:
Treat both conditions

Step 3: Psychological or pharmacologic intervention
Provide written materials on the benefits and possible disadvantages of each treatment as both are proven equally effective
Patient preference must be considered

Psychological: Cognitive behavioral therapy, other behavioral therapies

Pharmacologic: See Figure 9.2.5

Sources: (1) Canadian Psychiatric Association clinical practice guidelines for the management of anxiety disorders. *Can J Psychiatry.* 2006;51(Suppl. 2):1S–92S. (2) National Institute for Health and Clinical Excellence (2011) [Generalized anxiety disorder and panic disorder (with or without agoraphobia) in adults]. [113] London: National Institute for Health and Clinical Excellence.

FIGURE 9.2.5 Pharmacotherapy for Panic Disorder with or without Agoraphobia

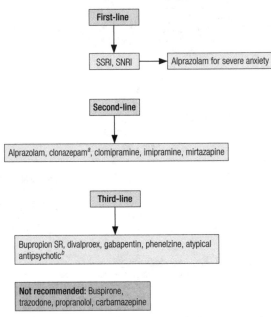

Source: Canadian Psychiatric Association clinical practice guidelines for the management of anxiety disorders. *Can J Psychiatry*. 2006;51(Suppl. 2):1S–92S.

[a]Short-term adjunctive clonazepam at the initiation of treatment can lead to an increased rapid response

[b]Consider referral to mental-health specialist.

FIGURE 9.2.6 Pharmacotherapy for Panic Disorder Treatment Resistance

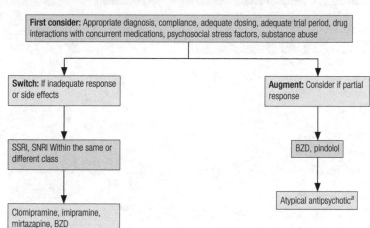

Sources: (1) World Federation of Societies of Biological Psychiatry (WFSBP) guidelines for the pharmacological treatment of anxiety, obsessive-compulsive and post-traumatic stress disorders—first revision. *World J Biol Psychiatry*. 2008;9(4):248–312. (2) Canadian Psychiatric Association clinical practice guidelines for the management of anxiety disorders. *Can J Psychiatry*. 2006;51(Suppl. 2):1S–92S.
^aConsider referral to mental-health specialist.

TABLE 9.2.7 Antidepressant Dosing for Anxiety Disorders

Generic Name	Trade Name	GAD Initial Dose (mg/day)	GAD Dosage Range (mg/day)	PD Initial Dose (mg/day)	PD Dosage Range (mg/day)
SSRIs					
Citalopram[a]	Celexa	20	20–60[b]	20	20–60[b]
Escitalopram	Lexapro	5–10	10–20	5–10	10–20
Fluoxetine[a]	Prozac	20	20–80	20	20–80
Fluvoxamine[a]	Luvox	50	100–300 divided BID	50	100–300 divided BID
Paroxetine[a]	Paxil	20	20–50	10	10–60
Sertraline[a]	Zoloft	50	50–200	50	50–200
SNRIs					
Duloxetine	Cymbalta	30–60	60, max 120	30–60	60, max 120
Venlafaxine XR[a]	Effexor XR	37.5	37.5–225	37.5	37.5–225
TCAs					
Clomipramine[a]	Anafranil	25	25–75	25	25–75
Imipramine[a]	Tofranil	25	75–150	25	75–150
MAOI					
Phenelzine[a]	Nardil	15 × 4 days	60–90 divided TID	15 × 4 days	60–90 divided TID
Other Antidepressants					
Bupropion SR[a]	Wellbutrin SR	100 BID SR 150 XL	300 SR divided BID	100 BID SR 150 XL	300 SR divided BID
Bupropion XL	Wellbutrin XL		300 XL		300 XL
Mirtazapine[a]	Remeron	15 QHS	15–45 QHS	15 QHS	15–45 QHS

Sources: (1) Micromedex® Healthcare Series [Internet database]. Greenwood Village, Colo: Thomson Reuters (Healthcare) Inc. (2) Canadian Psychiatric Association clinical practice guidelines for the management of anxiety disorders. *Can J Psychiatry.* 2006;51(Suppl. 2):1S–92S. (3) World Federation of Societies of Biological Psychiatry (WFSBP) guidelines for the pharmacological treatment of anxiety, obsessive-compulsive and post-traumatic stress disorders—first revision. *World J Biol Psychiatry.* 2008;9(4):248–312. (4) National Institute for Health and Clinical Excellence (2011) [Generalized anxiety disorder and panic disorder (with or without agoraphobia) in adults]. [113] London: National Institute for Health and Clinical Excellence.
[a]Generic formulations available.
[b]FDA guidelines do not recommend doses greater than 40 mg/daily.

TABLE 9.2.8 Other Medications for Anxiety Disorders

Generic Name	Trade Name	GAD Initial Dose (mg/day)	GAD Dosage Range (mg/day)	PD Initial Dose (mg/day)	PD Dosage Range (mg/day)
Gabapentin[a]	Neurontin	—	—	300 TID	900–3600 divided TID
Pregabalin	Lyrica	75 BID	200–450 divided BID or TID	—	—
Buspirone[a]	Buspar	5 TID or 7.5 BID	20–30 divided BID or TID Max 60	Not recommended	Not recommended

Sources: (1) Micromedex® Healthcare Series [Internet database]. Greenwood Village, Colo: Thomson Reuters (Healthcare) Inc. (2) Canadian Psychiatric Association clinical practice guidelines for the management of anxiety disorders. Can J Psychiatry 2006;51(Suppl. 2):1S–92S. (3) World Federation of Societies of Biological Psychiatry (WFSBP) guidelines for the pharmacological treatment of anxiety, obsessive-compulsive and post-traumatic stress disorders—first revision. World J Biol Psychiatry. 2008;9(4):248–312. (4) Bech P. Dose-response relationship of pregabalin in patients with generalized anxiety disorder. A pooled analysis of four placebo-controlled trials. Pharmacopsychiatry. 2007;40:163–168.
[a]Generic formulations available

TABLE 9.2.9 Benzodiazepines for Anxiety Disorders[a,b]

Generic Name	Trade Name	Initial Dose (mg/day)	Dosage Range (mg/day)	T_{max} (h)	Elimination ½ Life (Parent Drug) (h)	Active Metabolite
Alprazolam	Xanax Xanax XR	0.25 TID (IR) 0.5 (XR)	0.5–1 TID, max 4 0.5–1 XR	1–2	12–15	No
Clonazepam	Klonopin	0.25 BID	0.5–1 BID/TID, max 4	1–4	5–30	No
Diazepam	Valium	2 BID	2–10 BID, max 40	0.5–2	20–80	Yes
Lorazepam	Ativan	1 BID/TID	2 BID/TID, max 10	2–4	10–20	No
Oxazepam	Serax	10 TID/QID	10–30 TID/QID	2–4	5–20	No

Sources: Micromedex® Healthcare Series [Internet database]. Greenwood Village, Colo: Thomson Reuters (Healthcare) Inc.
[a]Taper slowly to avoid withdrawal symptoms, use lowest effective dose, tolerance may occur.
[b]Rebound anxiety may occur with short-acting agents (e.g., alprazolam).

TABLE 9.2.10 Preferred Medications in Special Populations

Population	Medication	Dose	Comments
Pregnancy: First trimester	Fluoxetine, sertraline, TCAs	Normal dosing	Avoid paroxetine and bupropion
Pregnancy: Second trimester	Fluoxetine, sertraline, TCAs	Normal dosing	Slight increased risk of pulmonary hypertension reported with SSRI use
Pregnancy: Third trimester	Fluoxetine, sertraline, TCAs	Possible dose increase	May require increased dose due to changes in drug metabolism and volume of distribution
Breastfeeding	Paroxetine, sertraline, nortriptyline	Normal dosing	Undetectable plasma levels in breastfed infants
Elderly	SSRIs		
	Citalopram, escitalopram, sertraline	Start at lowest possible dose Citalopram ≤20 mg in elderly	Negligible anticholinergic side effects and drug interactions
	BZDs		
	Lorazepam, oxazepam, temazepam	Lorazepam: 1–2 mg divided BID/TID	Use BZDs cautiously in elderly due to risk of falls and increased confusion
		Oxazepam: 10–15 mg TID/QID	

Sources: (1) Yonkers KA, Wisner KL, Stewart DE, et al. The management of depression during pregnancy: a report from the American Psychiatric Association and the American College of Obstetricians and Gynecologists. *Gen Hosp Psychiatry.* 2009;31:403–413. (2) Micromedex® Healthcare Series [Internet database]. Greenwood Village, Colo: Thomson Reuters (Healthcare) Inc.

FIGURE 9.3.1 Evaluation and Management of Insomnia

Initial assessment: Reported difficulty initiating or maintaining sleep; wakingup too early or sleep that is nonrestorative despite adequate opportunities and circumstance for sleep and includes at least 1 daytime impairment (fatigue, concentration or memory impairment, mood changes or irritability, loss of motivation or energy, worries about loss of sleep, errors at work or while driving, headaches or GI upset in response to lost sleep)

↓

Identify comorbid conditions and medications
- Identify and treat underlying sleep disorders (restless leg, obstructive sleep apnea) or medical, psychiatric, and substance abuse conditions associated with insomnia (see "Conditions Associated with Insomnia" box)
- Identify and remove substances or medications, which may interfere with sleep
  a. Alcohol, α-antagonists, α-agonists, β-agonists, β-blockers, caffeine, diuretics, nasal decongestants, SSRIs, steroids, stimulants

↓

Nonpharmacologic therapy (Use alone or with pharmacologic therapy)
- Sleep hygiene: Keep a regular schedule, eat a healthy diet, perform regular exercise, have a quiet sleep environment, avoid napping, limit caffeine, nicotine, alcohol, or excessive fluids near bedtime, avoid stimulating activities before bedtime
- Stimulus control: Keep a regular schedule, go to bed only when sleepy, use the bed only for sleep/sex, leave bed if unable to sleep after 20 min try relaxing activity (i.e., reading) until drowsy then go back to bed, repeat as necessary, avoid clock-checking
- Refer to therapist if available for relaxation therapy, cognitive behavioral therapy

Conditions associated with insomnia:
Cardiovascular: Angina, CHF, dyspnea, dysrhythmia
Endocrine: Hypo/hyperthyroidism, diabetes
GI: GERD, PUD, IBS, colitis
GU: Incontinence, BPH, cystitis
MSK: Arthritis, fibromyalgia, kyphosis
Neuro: Dementia, stroke, seizure, headache, migraine, neuropathy, chronic pain
Pulmonary: Asthma, COPD
Psychiatric: Depression, anxiety, mania, substance abuse/withdrawal
Reproductive: Pregnancy, menopause

(Continued)

FIGURE 9.3.1 Evaluation and Management of Insomnia *(Continued)*

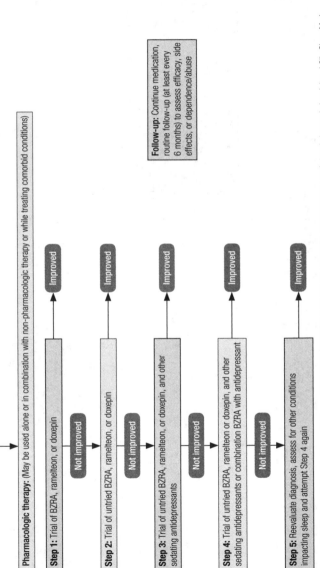

Pharmacologic therapy: (May be used alone or in combination with non-pharmacologic therapy or while treating comorbid conditions)

Step 1: Trial of BZRA, ramelteon, or doxepin

Step 2: Trial of untried BZRA, ramelteon, or doxepin

Step 3: Trial of untried BZRA, ramelteon, or doxepin, and other sedating antidepressants

Step 4: Trial of untried BZRA, ramelteon or doxepin, and other sedating antidepressants or combination BZRA with antidepressant

Step 5: Reevaluate diagnosis, assess for other conditions impacting sleep and attempt Step 4 again

Not improved

Improved

Follow-up: Continue medication, routine follow-up (at least every 6 months) to assess efficacy, side effects, or dependence/abuse

Source: Schutte-Rodin S, Broch L, Buysse D, Dorsey C, Sateia M. Clinical guideline for the evaluation and management of chronic insomnia in adults. *J Clin Sleep Med.* 2008;4(5):487–504.

TABLE 9.3.2 Drug Products and Dosing for Insomnia

Name	Availability	Dose (mg QHS)	T1/2 (h)	Comments	Adverse Effects/ Precautions
BZD					
Diazepam (Valium)	Generic T: 2, 5, 10 mg S: 5 mg/mL	A: 5–10	50–100	Long T1/2—Carry-over effects	Respiratory depression (avoid in comorbid OSA, COPD, or opiates) CNS depression (may impair abilities, increase fall risk, avoid with alcohol and CNS depressants)
Estazolam (Prosom)	Generic T: 1, 2 mg	A: 1–2 E: 0.5	10–24		Behavioral changes, sleep-related activities (such as driving, cooking, phone calls while sleeping), amnesia
Flurazepam (Dalmane)	Generic C: 15, 30 mg	A: 15–30 E: 15	40–114	Long T1/2—Carry-over effects	Dependence (withdrawal symptoms possible after 2 weeks, may require taper before discontinuation)
Lorazepam (Ativan)	Generic T: 0.5, 1, 2 mg S: 2 mg/mL	A: 2–4	10–20	No active metabolites	Abuse potential (all benzos are controlled (C-IV), avoid in hx of substance abuse)
Temazepam (Restoril)	Generic C: 7.5, 15, 22.5, 30 mg	A: 15–30 E: 7.5	10–40	No active metabolites	Not recommended for long-term use due to risk of dependence
Triazolam (Halcion)	Generic T: 0.125, 0.25 mg	A: 0.25–0.5 E: 0.125–0.25	2.3	Short T1/2 may cause rebound anxiety	

(Continued)

TABLE 9.3.2 Drug Products and Dosing for Insomnia *(Continued)*

Name	Availability	Dose (mg QHS)	T1/2 (h)	Comments	Adverse Effects/ Precautions
BZRA "Z Drugs"					
Eszopiclone (Lunesta)	Brand only T: 1, 2, 3 mg	A: 2–3 E: 1–2	6	"Z Drugs" are preferred over BZDs due to ↓risk of dependence/abuse	Respiratory depression (avoid in comorbid OSA, COPD, or opiates)
Zaleplon (Sonata)	Generic C: 5, 10 mg	A: 10–20 E: 5	1	Both eszopiclone and zolpidem have been shown safe and effective for up to 6 months cf nightly use	CNS depression (may impair mental/physical abilities, increase fall risk, avoid with alcohol, avoid with other CNS depressants)
Zolpidem (Ambien)	Generic Tabs only T: 5, 10 mg SL: 5, 10 mg Spray: 8.2 g	A: 10 E: 5	2.5	Zaleplon and zolpidem are ideal for sleep initiation, zolpidem CR able to be used for sleep maintenance	Behavioral changes, sleep-related activities (such as driving, cooking, phone calls while sleeping), amnesia
Zolpidem Controlled-Release (Ambien CR)	No generic T: 6.25, 12.5 mg	A: 12.5 E: 6.25	2.5		Abuse potential (Lower risk than with benzos but all Z Drugs are controlled (C-IV), avoid with hx of substance abuse)
Melatonin Agonists					
Ramelteon (Rozerem)	Brand only T: 8 mg	A: 8	1–2.5	Not controlled Approved for sleep maintenance	Behavioral changes, sleep-related activities (such as driving, cooking, phone calls while sleeping), changes in reproductive hormones (decreased libido or change in menses)
Sedating Antidepressants					
Doxepin (Silenor)	Brand only T: 3, 6 mg	A: 6 E: 3	15–31		Contraindicated with MAOIs or glaucoma and severe urinary retention CNS depressant, behavioral changes, sleep-related activities (such as driving, cooking, phone calls while sleeping)
Amitriptyline (Elavil)	Generic	A: 25–50 E: 10–25	9–27		Anticholinergic, orthostasis, EKG changes, lowers seizure threshold
Mirtazapine (Remeron)	Generic	A: 15 G: 7.5	20–40		Weight gain, hyperlipidemia,
Trazodone (Desyrel)	Generic	A: 25–200	7–10		Orthostasis, priapism, QTc prolongation, hyponatremia, dizziness, blurry vision, dry mouth

FIGURE 9.3.3 Assessment and Management of Narcolepsy

Initial assessment:

Narcolepsy with cataplexy
- Excessive daytime sleepiness for the past 3 months
- Definite history of cataplexy (Sudden bilateral loss of postural muscle tone occurs in association with intense emotion)
- May be confirmed by polysomnography or CSF-hypocretin-1 level <110 pg/mL

Narcolepsy without cataplexy
- Excessive daytime sleepiness for the past 3 months
- *Must be* confirmed by polysomnography

Narcolepsy caused by a medical condition
- Excessive daytime sleeping for the past 3 months
- Significant underlying medical or neurologic condition accounts for daytime sleepiness
- Definite history of cataplexy is present or if no cataplexy present, then confirmation by polysomnography or CSF-hypocretin-1 level <110 pg/mL

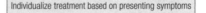

Individualize treatment based on presenting symptoms

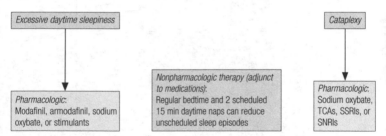

Excessive daytime sleepiness

Pharmacologic:
Modafinil, armodafinil, sodium oxybate, or stimulants

Nonpharmacologic therapy (adjunct to medications):
Regular bedtime and 2 scheduled 15 min daytime naps can reduce unscheduled sleep episodes

Cataplexy

Pharmacologic:
Sodium oxybate, TCAs, SSRIs, or SNRIs

Source: Morgenthaler TI, Kapur VK, Brown TM, et al. Practice parameters for the treatment of narcolepsy and other hypersomnias of central origin. *Sleep.* 2007;30:1705–1711.

TABLE 9.3.4 Drug Dosing for Narcolepsy[a]

Drug	Availability	Dose	Adverse Effects	Comments
Stimulants				
Dextroamphetamine salts (Adderall)	Generic T: 5, 10, 15, 20, 30 mg	10 mg/day, ↑ by 10 mg/week to max 60 mg/day divided BID-TID	Psychosis, ↑HR, ↑BP, anorexia, insomnia, irritability, headache, dry mouth, abdominal pain, dysphoria	*FDA-approved for narcolepsy* Controlled (C-II) Avoid in hx of substance abuse
Methylphenidate (Ritalin)	Generic T: 5, 10, 20 mg	10 mg daily (↑ by 10 mg/week) up to 60 mg/day divided BID-TID		
Armodafinil (Nuvigil)	Brand only T: 50, 150, 250 mg	150 mg–250 mg daily	Headache, anxiety, nausea, dry mouth, diarrhea, asthenia, insomnia, ↑HR	*FDA-approved for narcolepsy* Controlled (C-IV)
Modafinil (Provigil)	Brand only T: 100, 200 mg	Initially 200–400 mg/day, add 200 mg at noon if residual sleepiness		
Sodium oxybate (Xyrem)	Brand only 500 mg/mL	4.6–9 g divided evenly QHS and then 2.5–4 h later	Avoid activities requiring mental alertness for 6 h, confusion, dizziness, nausea, enuresis	*FDA-approved for narcolepsy* Controlled (C-III) Prescribers must be registered with Xyrem Program

[a]SSRIs, SNRIs and TCAs may all be used for cataplexy at standard doses, see table 9.1.2 for dosing.

FIGURE 9.3.5 Obstructive Sleep Apnea Assessment and Treatment Algorithm

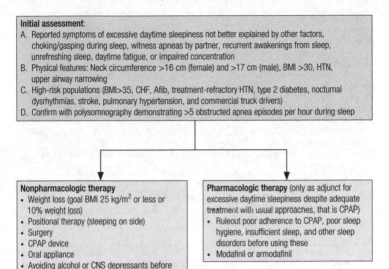

Initial assessment:
A. Reported symptoms of excessive daytime sleepiness not better explained by other factors, choking/gasping during sleep, witness apneas by partner, recurrent awakenings from sleep, unrefreshing sleep, daytime fatigue, or impaired concentration
B. Physical features: Neck circumference >16 cm (female) and >17 cm (male), BMI >30, HTN, upper airway narrowing
C. High-risk populations (BMI>35, CHF, Afib, treatment-refractory HTN, type 2 diabetes, nocturnal dysrhythmias, stroke, pulmonary hypertension, and commercial truck drivers)
D. Confirm with polysomnography demonstrating >5 obstructed apnea episodes per hour during sleep

Nonpharmacologic therapy
- Weight loss (goal BMI 25 kg/m² or less or 10% weight loss)
- Positional therapy (sleeping on side)
- Surgery
- CPAP device
- Oral appliance
- Avoiding alcohol or CNS depressants before bed (opiates/benzos)

Pharmacologic therapy (only as adjunct for excessive daytime sleepiness despite adequate treatment with usual approaches, that is CPAP)
- Ruleout poor adherence to CPAP, poor sleep hygiene, insufficient sleep, and other sleep disorders before using these
- Modafinil or armodafinil

Source: Epstein LJ, Kristo D, Strollo PJ, et al. Clinical guidelines for the evaluation, management and long-term care of obstructive sleep apnea in adults. *J Clin Sleep Med.* 2009;5:263–276.

TABLE 9.3.6 Drug Dosing for Obstructive Sleep Apnea

Drug	Availability	Dose	Adverse Effects	Comments
Armodafinil (Nuvigil)	Brand only T: 50, 150, 250 mg	150 mg–250 mg daily	Headache, anxiety, nausea, dry mouth, diarrhea, asthenia, insomnia, ↑HR	FDA-approved for OSA Controlled (C-IV)
Modafinil (Provigil)	Brand only T: 100, 200 mg	200 mg—400 mg daily		

FIGURE 9.4.1 Assessment and Management of RLS Algorithm

Initial assessment:
Diagnosis
Essential criteria (all must be present): Urge to move (generally with uncomfortable sensation) starting in the legs, Onset or exacerbation during periods of rest/inactivity, Relief with movement or stretching, Sx occur or are worse in the evening or night
Supportive criteria (used to help confirm dx): 3–5× more likely among first-degree relatives; Most people with RLS show response to dopamine agonists; periodic limb movement occurs in 85% of cases
Associated features: Age of onset >50 sx are abrupt and severe, if <50 then sx are insidious, sleep disturbances are common, physical exam is normal and does not contribute to diagnosis except to ruleout other disorders
Labs: Obtain iron studies (ferritin, %iron saturation), kidney function, folic acid, b12, and thyroid function to rule out secondary causes or mimicking disorders
Identify contributing medications: Antidepressants (except bupropion), antipsychotics, metoclopramide, prochlorperazine, promethazine

Iron deficiency: If ferritin<25 µg/L or iron saturation <20%, then initiate $FeSO_4$ 325 mg TID with vitamin C 100–200 mg TID, obtain follow-up iron studies after 3–4 months; if ferritin >50 µg/L and iron sturation >20%, then $FeSO_4$ can be discontinued

Medications: If on medication potentially worsening RLS, consider discontinuing or switching to a different medication; if not possible, then treat RLS with medications (see Pharmacologic Therapy)

Nonpharmacologic treatment (For use with/without pharmacologic therapy)
• Trial of abstinence from caffeine, alcohol, and nicotine or restrict use after 3:00 PM
• Mentally alerting activities (video games, conversation, painting or puzzles) during time of boredom when symptoms may arise
• Schedule sedentary activities early in the day and active activities later

Pharmacologic therapy

Intermittent RLS—Not occurring daily

Levodopa/carbidopa, dopamine agonist, or tramadol

Daily RLS

Dopamine agonists, gabapentin, or tramadol

Refractory daily RLS
1. Inadequate response despite adequate dose
2. Loss of response over time
3. Intolerable adverse effects
4. Augmentation: worsening of sx earlier in the day

Switch to untried dopamine agonist, gabapentin, tramadol, oxycodone, or try combination of dopamine agonist with gabapentin, tramadol, or oxycodone

Source: Rye DM, Adler CH, Allen RP, et al. RLS medical bulletin: a publication for healthcare providers. Restless Legs Syndrome Foundation. 2005. www.rls.org. Accessed November 20, 2011.

TABLE 9.4.2 Drug Dosing for RLS

Drug	Availability	Dose	Adverse Effects	Comments
Dopamine Agonists				
Carbidopa/levodopa (Sinemet, Sinemet CR)	Generic T: 25/100	25/100 QHS	Orthostasis, dyskinesias, compulsive gambling, binge eating, hypersexuality, rebound (early morning RLS), augmentation Earlier morning RLS symptoms	Off-label for RLS IR can be used PRN for plane rides, movie theaters, and midnight awakenings Not preferred for daily RLS due to rebound/ augmentation Do not take with protein-foods do to ↑ absorption
Pramipexole (Mirapex)	Generic T: 0.25, 0.5, 1, 1.5 mg	0.125 mg × 3 days, double dose every 4–7 days, usual cose 0.5 mg/day (max 2 mg/day)	Nausea, headache, orthostasis, dyskinesias, compulsive gambling, binge eating, hypersexuality, rebound (early morning RLS), augmentation (earlier RLS symptoms)	Both FDA-approved IR formulation for RLS Give 2–3 h before bed Give earlier in the day if augmentation occurs Convert from ropinirole 3:1 ratio
Ropinirole (Requip)	Generic T: 0.25, 0.5, 1, 2, 3, 4 mg	0.25 mg × 3 days, then 0.5 × 3 days then ↑ by 0.5 mg/week to usual dose 2 mg/day (max 4 mg/day)		
Anticonvulsants				
Gabapentin (Neurontin)	Generic C: 100, 300, 400 mg	Initial 300 mg, titrate every 2 weeks (300–1800 mg/day),	CNS depression, dizziness, sommolence, ataxia, peripheral edema,	Off-label for RLS Take 2 h before bedtime Split dose >600 mg into late afternoon and evening or 1/3 at noon and 2/3 at 8 PM
Opioid analgesics				
Tramadol (Ultram)	Generic T: 50, 100, 200 mg	50–150 mg QHS	Constipation, nausea. flushing, dizziness, sommolence, insomnia,	Off-label for RLS
Oxycodone (Roxicet)	Generic T: 5, 10, 15 mg	5–15 mg QHS	Respiratory depression, CNS depression, dizziness, nausea. constipation, abuse/dependence	Off-label for RLS Controlled (C-II)

ABBREVIATIONS

DSG	Desogestrel	NGM	Norgestimate
DSP	Drospirenone	NTE	Norethindrone
EE	Ethinyl estradiol	NTE ac	Norethindrone acetate
HFI	Hormone-free interval	OCs	Oral contraceptives
IUD	Intrauterine device	VTE	Venous thromboembolism
LVN	Levonorgestrel		

TABLE 10.1.1 Marketed OC Products

Original Brand Name[a]	Branded Generic Names[b]	Estrogen Component	Progestin Component	Regimen[c]	Comments
Alesse	Aviane-28, Lessina, Lutera, Sronyx	EE 20 μg	LVN 0.1 mg	27/7 HFI	Monophasic
Loestrin Fe 1/20	Junel Fe 1.5/20, Microgestin Fe 1/20	EE 20 μg	NTE ac 1 mg	21/7 HFI	Monophasic; HFI contains ferrous fumarate
Nordette	Levora, Portia 28	EE 30 μg	LVN 0.15 mg	21/7 HFI	Monophasic
Lo/Ovral	Low-Ogestrel, Cryselle 28	EE 30 mg	Norgestrel 0.3 mg	21/7 HFI	Monophasic
Loestrin Fe 1.5/30	Junel 1.5/30, Microgestin Fe 1.5/30	EE 30 μg	NTE ac 1.5 mg	21/7 HFI	Monophasic; HFI contains ferrous fumarate
Desogen, Ortho-Cept	Apri, Reclipsen, Solia	EE 30 μg	DSG 0.15 mg	21/7 HFI	Monophasic
Yasmin	Ocella, Zarah	EE 30 μg	DSP 3 mg	21/7 HFI	Monophasic
Demulen	Kelnor 1/35, Zovia 1/35	EE 35 μg	Ethynodiol diacetate 1 mg	21/7 HFI	Monophasic
Ortho-Cyclen	MonoNessa, Previfem, Sprintec	EE 35 μg	NGM 0.25 mg	21/7 HFI	Monophasic
Ortho Novum 1/50	Norinyl 1 + 50, Necon 1/50	Mestranol 50 μg	NTE 1 mg	21/7 HFI	Monophasic; mestranol is converted into EE
Ovcon-35	Balziva, Zenchent	EE 35 μg	NTE 0.4 mg	21/7 HFI	Monophasic
Femcon Fe Chewable	Zeosa, Generess Fe	EE 35 μg	NTE 0.4 mg	21/7 HFI	Monophasic; HFI contains ferrous fumarate; chewable
Modicon-28	Brevicon-28, Necon 0.5/35; Nortrel 0.5/35	EE 35 μg	NTE 0.5 mg	21/7 HFI	Monophasic
Ortho-Novum 1/35	Necon 1/35; Norinyl 1 + 35; Nortrel 1/35	EE 35 μg	NTE 1 mg	21/7 HFI	Monophasic
Ovcon-50		EE 50 μg	NTE 1 mg	21/7 HFI	Monophasic; high dose

(Continued)

TABLE 10.1.1 Marketed OC Products (Continued)

Original Brand Name[a]	Branded Generic Name[b]	Estrogen Component	Progestin Component	Regimen[c]	Comments
Ovral	Ogestrel	EE 50 μg	Norgestrel 0.5 mg	21/7 HFI	Monophasic; high dose
Demulen 1/50	Zovia 1/50	EE 50 μg	Ethynodiol diacetate 1 mg	21/7 HFI	Monophasic; high dose
Mircette	Azurette, Kariva 28	EE 20 μg	DSG 0.15 mg	21/2 plcb/5 EE 10 μg	Biphasic
Ortho-Novum 10/11	Necon 10/11	EE 35 μg	NTE 0.5 mg × 10 days; 1 mg × 11 days	10/11	Biphasic
Estrostep Fe	Tilia Fe, Tri-Legest Fe 28	EE 20 μg × 5 days; 30 μg × 7 days; 10 μg × 9 days	NTE ac 1 mg × 21 days	5/7/9/7 HFI	Triphasic; HFI contains ferrous fumarate
Ortho Tri-Cyclen Lo	Tri Lo Sprintec	EE 25 μg	NGM 0.18 mg × 7 days; 0.215 mg × 7 days; 0.25 mg × 7 days	7/7/7/7 HFI	Triphasic
Cyclessa	Caziant, Cesia, Velivet	EE 25 μg	DSG 0.1 mg × 7 days; 0.125 mg × 7 days; 0.15 mg × 7 days	7/7/7/7 HFI	Triphasic
Triphasil	Enpresse 28, Trivora	EE 30 μg × 6 days; 40 μg × 5 days; 30 μg × 10 days	LVN 0.05 mg × 6 days; 0.075 mg × 5 days; 0.125 mg × 10 days	6/5/10/7 HFI	Triphasic
Ortho Tri-Cyclen	TriNessa, Tri-Previfem, Tri-Sprintec	EE 35 μg	NGM 0.18 mg × 7 days; 0.215 mg × 7 days; 0.25 mg × 7 days	7/7/7/7 HFI	Triphasic
Tri-Norinyl	Aranelle, Leena	EE 35 μg	NTE 0.5 mg × 7 days; 1 mg × 9 days; 0.5 mg × 5 days	7/9/5/7 HFI	Triphasic
Ortho-Novum 7/7/7	Nortrel 7/7/7, Necon 7/7/7	EE 35 μg	NTE 0.5 mg × 7 days; 0.75 mg × 7 days; 1 rng × 7 days	7/7/7/7 HFI	Triphasic

		Estradiol valerate	Dienogest none × 2 days; 2 mg × 5 days; 3 mg × 17 days; none × 4 days	2/5/17/2/2 HFI	Four phasic
Natazia		Estradiol valerate 3 mg × 2 days; 2 mg × 22 days; 1 mg × 2 days; 2 day HFI	Dienogest none × 2 days; 2 mg × 5 days; 3 mg × 17 days; none × 4 days	2/5/17/2/2 HFI	Four phasic
Lo Loestrin Fe		EE 10 µg × 26 days	NTE ac 1 mg × 24 cays	24/2/2 HFI	Extended cycle; HFI contains ferrous fumarate
Loestrin-24 Fe		EE 20 µg × 24 days	NTE ac 1 mg × 24 days	24/4 HFI	Extended cycle; HFI contains ferrous fumarate
LoSeasonique		EE 20 µg × 84 days; 10 µg × 7 days	LVN 0.1 mg × 84 days	84/7	Extended cycle with low-dose EE last 7 days
Seasonale	Jolessa, Quasense, Introvale	EE 30 µg × 84 days	LVN 0.15 mg × 84 days	84/7 HFI	Extended cycle
Seasonique	Camrese, Amethia	EE 30 µg × 84 days; 10 µg × 7 days	LVN 0.15 mg × 84 days	84/7	Extended cycle with low-dose EE last 7 days
Yaz	Gianvi	EE 20 µg × 24 days	DSP 3 mg × 24 days	24/4 HFI	Extended cycle
Beyaz		EE 20 µg × 24 days	DSP 3 mg × 24 days	24/4 HFI	Extended cycle; each tab also contains levomefolate 0.451 mg
Lybrel	Amethyst	EE 20 µg	LVN 90 µg	28 (no HFI)	Continuous cycle

Sources: (1) Comparison of oral contraceptives: a summary. *Pharmacist's Letter/Prescriber's Letter* 2007;23(12):231207 (full update June 2010). Watson Pharmaceuticals. (2) http://www.watson.com/products/product-database-detail.asp?group=business&c=18. Accessed August 4, 2011. (3) Teva Pharmaceuticals. http://www.tevausa.com/default.aspx?pageid=76&TherapeuticCategory=Contraceptives Accessed August 8, 2011.

aSome original products are no longer available

bMay not contain all current products; products may be discontinued. Not all products are AB rated for substitution.

cDays of each dose per pillpack

TABLE 10.1.2 Progestin-Only OCs[a]

Original Brand Names	Branded Generic Names	Progestin Component
Micronor, Nor-QD	Camila, Erin, Heather, Jolivette, Nora-BE	NTE 0.35 mg × 28 days

[a]American College of Obstetrics and Gynecology considers progestin-only oral contraceptives to be safer than combined contraceptives for the following situations: Migraine headaches, especially those with focal neurologic signs; cigarette smoking or obesity in women older than 35 years; history of thromboembolic disease; hypertension in women with vascular disease or older than 35 years; systemic lupus erythematosus with vascular disease, nephritis, or antiphospholipid antibodies; less than 3 weeks postpartum; hypertriglyceridemia; CAD; CHF; cerebrovascular disease (ACOG Practice Bulletin, Number 73,2006 *Obstet Gynecol.* 2006;107(6):1453–1472).

TABLE 10.1.3 Initiating OC Therapy

Day 1 Start	Take first active tablet within first 24 h of menses	No backup contraception required but a conservative recommendation is to use backup contraception for 7 days
Sunday Start	Take first active tablet on the first Sunday after menses starts	Use a nonhormonal method of contraception for first 7 days
Quick Start	Take first active tablet on day of availability (often in the physician's office), regardless of menstrual cycle day. Rule out pregnancy if in question.	Use backup contraception for first 7 days, or more conservatively, until next menses
Postpartum (non-breastfeeding women)	No combined hormonal contraceptives for 21 days after delivery.	
	Without VTE risk factors, OCs may be initiated days 21–42 after delivery.	Risk of ovulation can occur as early as 25 days postpartum; nonhormonal contraception may be needed before initiating OCs and during first 7 days depending on sexual activity
	With VTE risk factors (such as previous VTE, cesarean delivery), OCs may be initiated after 42 days after delivery.	Nonhormonal contraception may be needed before initiating OCs and during first 7 days depending on sexual activity

TABLE 10.1.4 Managing Missed OC Tablets

- During weeks 1 and 2, if 1 tablet is missed, take as soon as it is remembered. This may result in taking 2 tablets at one time (no backup contraception required)
- During weeks 1 and 2, if 2 tablets are missed, then take 2 tablets at a time for the next 2 days (use backup contraception for the next 7 days)
- For missed tablets later in a pillpack, refer to product labeling, but the general recommendation is to begin a new pillpack and use backup contraception
- For extended cycle OCs and OCs that contain more than 1 phase, refer to product labeling

TABLE 10.1.5 Hormonal Components of OC Products

Estrogens

EE—estrogen in almost all OCs

Mestranol—hepatic metabolism to EE

Estradiol valerate—esterified form of estradiol that is hydrolyzed to estradiol

Progestins

19-nortestosterone derivatives

Estranes (slight estrogenic activity)—NTE, NTE ac, ethynodiol diacetate

Gonanes—LVN, norgestrel, NGM, DSG, dienogest (mild antiandrogenic activity)

Spironolactone derivative—DSP (progestogenic, antiandrogenic, and antimineralocorticoid activity)

Sources: (1) Fritz MA, Speroff L. *Clinical Gynecologic Endocrinology and Infertility* 8th ed. Philadelphia, PA: Lippincott Williams and Wilkins; 2011. http://ovidsp.tx.ovid.com/sp-3.4.1b/ovidweb.cgi. Accessed August 9, 2011.
(2) Lohr PA, Creinin MD. Oral contraceptives and breakthrough bleeding: what patients need to know. *J Fam Pract.* 2006;55(10):872–880.

TABLE 10.1.6 Emergency Contraceptives

Brand Name	Contains	Mechanism of Action	Regimen	Regulatory Status	Dosing Window
Plan B One-Step	1 LVN 1.5 mg tab	Alters ovulation	1 tab as soon as possible	By prescription for age < 17; OTC for age ≥17	Up to 72 h after unprotected intercourse
Next Choice	2 LVN 0.75 mg tabs	Alters ovulation	1 tab as soon as possible; 2nd tab 12 h later	By prescription for age <17; OTC for age ≥17	Up to 72 h after unprotected intercourse
Ella	1 ulipristal acetate 30 mg tab (may be repeated if patient vomits within 3 h of ingestion)	Progesterone agonist/antagonist that delays or inhibits ovulation (by preventing follicular rupture)	1 tab as soon as possible	Prescription	Up to 120 h after unprotected intercourse

TABLE 10.1.7 Contraception with Chronic Medical Problems

Condition	Concerns	Preferred Method of Contraception	Acceptable Alternatives	Avoid	Comments
Bariatric surgery	Reduced oral absorption of contraceptives with malabsorptive bariatric surgeries (Roux-en-Y bypass)	Agents that do not require oral absorption (note: no preference for restrictive-type procedures)		OCs	Vomiting after bariatric procedures may also reduce OC effectiveness
Breastfeeding	Estrogen may negatively affect the establishment of milk production and quantity	Progestin-only contraceptives	Estrogen-containing contraceptives after first postpartum month: Copper IUD (lower expulsion rate with early insertion (up to 72 h after delivery)		A neonate may be at risk due to exposure to steroid hormones with LVN-releasing IUD use during the first 4 weeks
Diabetes	Possible impaired glucose control and carbohydrate metabolism	*Without vascular disease:* Copper IUD *With vascular complications or diabetes >20 years:* Copper IUD	*Without vascular disease:* All types of contraceptives *With vascular complications or diabetes >20 years:* Oral progestin OCs, implants, LVN-releasing IUD	*With vascular complications or diabetes >20 years:* Estrogen-containing OCs, depot medroxyprogesterone	Depot medroxyprogesterone may have negative effects on lipid metabolism possibly affecting progression of nephropathy, retinopathy, and other vascular disease
Epilepsy	Some antiepileptic medications may induce hepatic enzymes and reduce serum concentrations of contraceptive hormones	*If taking lamotrigine:* All forms except estrogen-containing contraceptives (see Table 10.1.8) *If taking phenytoin, carbamazepine, barbiturates, primidone, topiramate, or oxcarbazepine:* Depot medroxyprogesterone or IUDs	*If taking phenytoin, carbamazepine, barbiturates, primidone, topiramate, or oxcarbazepine:* Implants	*If taking lamotrigine:* Estrogen-containing contraceptives *If taking phenytoin, carbamazepine, barbiturates, primidone, topiramate, or oxcarbazepine:* OCs (both types) Some experts recommend higher dose OCs instead (see Table 10.1.8)	Anticonvulsants that do not affect OC levels: Ethosuximide, gabapentin, levetiracetam, tiagabine, valproic acid, and zonisamide

		Not receiving anticoagulant therapy or for ≤3 months:	Not receiving anticoagulant therapy or for ≤3 months:	Not receiving anticoagulant therapy or for ≤3 months:	
Hypercoagulable conditions with history of deep venous thrombosis (DVT) or pulmonary embolism (PE)	Increased coagulability and risk of thromboembolism due to estrogen content	*Not receiving anticoagulant therapy or for ≤3 months:* Copper IUD *Taking anticoagulant therapy for at least 3 months:* All forms of contraception other than estrogen containing	*Not receiving anticoagulant therapy or for ≤3 months:* Progestin-only contraceptives	*Not receiving anticoagulant therapy or for ≤3 months:* Estrogen-containing contraceptives unless no current identifiable risk factors *Taking anticoagulant therapy for at least 3 months:* Estrogen-containing contraceptives (although some experts feel that this is an acceptable option)	Family history does not preclude any agents
Headache/ migraine	Estrogen-containing contraceptives may increase risk of stroke (migraine with aura)	*Nonmigraine headaches:* All forms *Migraines without aura:* Copper IUD or progestin-only OCs *Migraines with aura:* Copper IUD *Menstrual migraine:* Continuous or extended combined estrogen/progestin hormonal contraceptives	*Migraines without aura:* If younger than age 35, all others are acceptable. If 35 or older, all others except estrogen-containing contraceptives *Migraines with aura:* All others except estrogen-containing contraceptives	*Migraines without aura and age 35 or older:* Estrogen-containing contraceptives *Migraines with aura:* Estrogen-containing contraceptives	Women who develop migraine headaches (with or without aura) or have worsening headaches on estrogen-containing contraceptives should discontinue their use
Hyperlipidemia	Oral estrogen may increase triglycerides and progestins may increase LDL cholesterol	Copper IUD	Use estrogen/progestin-containing OCs with caution if total cholesterol, LDL, and/ or triglycerides are elevated. All others are acceptable.		Consider an OC with less androgenic progestin compared with more androgenic progestin Monitor fasting lipids in women with controlled dyslipidemias using a combination OC

(Continued)

TABLE 10.1.7 Contraception with Chronic Medical Problems (Continued)

Condition	Concerns	Preferred Method of Contraception	Acceptable Alternatives	Avoid	Comments
Hypertension	Estrogen may increase BP and increase risk of cardiovascular events in women with hypertension	*Adequately controlled BP or with SBP 140–159 mm Hg or DBP 90–99 mm Hg:* All except estrogen-containing contraceptives *SBP 160 mm Hg or greater or DBP 100 mm Hg or greater:* Copper IUD	*SBP 160 mm Hg or greater or DBP 100 mm Hg or greater:* Progestin-only OCs, implants, or LVN-releasing IUD	*Adequately controlled BP or with SBP 140–159 mm Hg or DBP 90–99 mm Hg:* Estrogen-containing contraceptives *SBP 160 mm Hg or greater or DBP 100 mm Hg or greater:* Estrogen-containing contraceptives and depot medroxyprogesterone	Cardiovascular risk may be greater if other conditions coexist (e.g., hyperlipidemia, obesity) If possible, control BP prior to initiating contraception and continue to monitor BP Concern about the possible negative effect of depot medroxyprogesterone on lipid metabolism and potential progression of nephropathy, retinopathy, or other vascular disease
Obesity	Obesity is an independent risk factor for VTE, and women who use combined estrogen/progestin OCs may have an increased risk of VTE. Conflicting reports of higher failure rates	*BMI ≤ 40:* All except contraceptive patch	Use the contraceptive patch with caution in women 90 kg or greater due to possible decreased efficacy		Some experts have suggested a high-dose estrogen OC in heavier women, while some experts suggest this increases the risk of thrombosis. Decreasing or eliminating the pill-free interval may be a better strategy in heavier women

Condition	Disease considerations				Comments
Rheumatoid arthritis	Estrogens and/or progestins may affect control of the disease. Depot medroxyprogesterone may increase risk of fractures.	All		Avoid depot medroxyprogesterone in women on long-term corticosteroid therapy	
Smoking	Older studies of combined OCs with 50 µg or more of estrogen demonstrated increased risk of myocardial infarction in women in their mid-30s or older	*Younger than 35:* All; *35 years or older:* All except estrogen-containing contraceptives		*35 years or older:* Estrogen-containing contraceptives	More recent data is conflicting regarding the increased risk of myocardial infarction with OCs containing <50 µg of estrogen
Stroke	Hormonal contraception can increase the risk of hypercoagulability and stroke	Copper IUD	LVN-releasing IUD	All others	Early studies of OCs and stroke used 50 µg of estrogen. Studies with lower doses have found conflicting information
Systemic lupus erythematosus	Increased risk of ischemic heart disease, stroke, and VTE especially in women with antiphospholipid antibodies	*Positive or unknown antiphospholipid antibodies:* Copper IUD; *Receiving immunosuppressive therapy (and antiphospholipid antibody negative):* Copper IUD	*Receiving immunosuppressive therapy (and antiphospholipid antibody negative):* All others	*Positive or unknown antiphospholipid antibodies;* All others	

Adapted with permission from Contraception for women with chronic medical conditions. Pharmacist's Letter/Prescriber's Letter 2011;27(3):270306. www.therapeuticresearch.com.

TABLE 10.1.8 Anti-infective, Antiviral, Antibiotic, and Anticonvulsant Drug Interactions with OCs

Drug Class	Generic Name	Decrease OC Efficacy?	Comments
Broad spectrum antibiotics	Various	Controversial; most evidence is anecdotal. A subset of women with lower hormonal concentrations may be more susceptible to pregnancy	Conservative thought is to use backup contraception during treatment course and at least 1 week after stopping antibiotic for short-term therapy, and for first 2 weeks of treatment course during long-term therapy
Anticonvulsants	Carbamazepine	Yes	Alternate method of contraception; some experts recommend a higher dose OC
	Phenobarbital	Yes	Alternate method of contraception; some experts recommend a higher dose OC
	Phenytoin	Yes	Alternate method of contraception; some experts recommend a higher dose OC
	Primidone	Yes	Alternate method of contraception; some experts recommend a higher dose OC
	Clonazepam	No	
	Ethosuximide	No	
	Valproate	No	
	Oxcarbazepine	Yes	Alternate method of contraception; some experts recommend a higher dose OC
	Felbamate	Yes	Alternate method of contraception; some experts recommend a higher dose OC
	Topiramate	Yes	At doses >200 mg/day
	Gabapentin	No	
	Lamotrigine	No	Lamotrigine may decrease the progestin plasma concentration by 10–19% (study was done with an EE/LVN OC); not clinically significant in most patients, except possibly with progestin-only OCs. The estrogen component can enhance the metabolism of lamotrigine and decrease serum concentrations by >50%. Concomitant use of lamotrigine and phenytoin, phenobarbital, primidone, or carbamazepine (in addition to an OC) do not require adjustment of lamotrigine maintenance dose
	Levetiracetam	No	
	Pregabalin	No	

	Tiagabine	No	
	Vigabatrin	No	
	Zonisamide	No	
	Lacosamide	No	
Anti-infectives	Rifampin	Yes	Backup method of contraception during use and 1 month following treatment
	Griseofulvin	Yes	Backup method of contraception
Antivirals			
Protease inhibitors	Amprenavir/Fosamprenavir	Yes	Backup method of contraception
	Atazanavir	No	Hormonal plasma concentrations increased; manufacturer recommends using lowest possible dose of OC
	Darunavir	Yes	Backup method of contraception
	Indinavir	No	
	Lopinavir/Ritonavir	Yes	Backup method of contraception
	Nelfinavir	Yes	Backup method of contraception
	Ritonavir	Yes	Backup method of contraception
	Tipranavir	Yes	Backup method of contraception

(Continued)

TABLE 10.1.8 **Anti-infective, Antiviral, Antibiotic, and Anticonvulsant Drug Interactions with OCs** *(Continued)*

Drug Class	Generic Name	Decrease OC Efficacy?	Comments
Non-nucleoside reverse transcriptase inhibitors	Efavirenz	No	Plasma concentrations of EE were increased in a small study; significance is not fully known
	Nevirapine	Yes	Backup method of contraception
Nucleoside and nucleotide reverse transcriptase inhibitors	Various	No	Not all agents have data, but are not expected to interact with OCs as they do not commonly affect liver enzymes such as CYP450
CCR5 antagonist	Maraviroc	No	

Sources: (1) Shenfield GM, Griffin JM. Clinical pharmacokinetics of contraceptive steroids. An update. *Clin Pharmacokinet.* 1991;20:15–37. (2) Oral contraceptive (OC) drug interactions. *Pharmacist's Letter/Prescriber's Letter* 2005;21(9):210903. (3) Johannsen LC, Patsalos PN. Drug interactions involving the new second and third generation antiepileptic drugs. *Expert Rev Neurother* 2010;10:119–140. (4) GlaxoSmithKline. Lamictal® (lamotrigine) tablets and chewable dispersible tablets prescribing information. Research Triangle Park; NC; 2011 Jul. (5) El-Ibiary SY, Cocohoba JM. Effects of HIV retrovirals on the pharmacokinetics of hormonal contraceptives. *Eur J Contracept Reprod Health Care.* 2008;13:123–132.

TABLE 10.1.9 Comparison of OC and Menopausal Hormone Therapy Contraindications

OCs	Menopausal Hormone Therapy
DVT/pulmonary embolism, active or history	DVT/pulmonary embolism, active or history
Cerebral vascular or coronary artery disease	Arterial thromboembolic disease (stroke, myocardial infarction)—active or recent
Known or suspected pregnancy	Known or suspected pregnancy
Known or suspected breast cancer	Known or suspected breast cancer
Endometrial carcinoma or other suspected estrogen-dependent neoplasia	Estrogen-dependent neoplasia
Undiagnosed abnormal genital bleeding	Undiagnosed abnormal genital bleeding
Hepatic adenomas or carcinomas or active liver disease	Liver dysfunction or disease
Cholestatic jaundice of pregnancy or jaundice with prior hormonal contraceptive use	
Smoking and age >35 years	
Diabetes with vascular involvement	
Headaches with focal neurological symptoms	
Uncontrolled hypertension	

Note: Not all contraindications are phrased exactly alike for each class of drug, although it generally follows class labeling; above is a summary based on multiple package inserts.

ABBREVIATIONS

ACCP	American College of Chest Physicians	LMWH	Low-molecular-weight heparin
APA	Antiphospholipid antibody syndrome	NCCN	National Comprehensive Cancer Network
CKD	Chronic kidney disease	PCC	Prothrombin complex concentrate
ESA	Erythropoietin-stimulating agent	PPI	Proton pump inhibitor
FFP	Fresh frozen plasma	VTE	Venous thromboembolism
HIT	Heparin-induced thrombocytopenia		
K/DOQI	The Kidney Disease Outcomes Quality Initiative		

TABLE 11.1.1 Iron Products for Treatment of Anemia

Drug	Dosing	Comments
Oral Iron		
Ferrous fumarate 200 mg (66 mg elemental) 325 mg (106 mg elemental)	• 150–200 mg elemental per day for most patients	• K/DOQI guidelines suggest 200 mg elemental per day for dialysis patients • Common adverse effects are constipation, diarrhea, nausea, vomiting, and darkened stools
Ferrous gluconate 246 mg (28 mg elemental) 300 mg (34 mg elemental) 325 mg (36 mg elemental)		• Food, PPIs, and antacids decrease absorption • Taking with a vitamin C source (orange juice or 50–100 mg ascorbic acid tablet) can improve tolerability and absorption (*Hum Nutr Appl Nutr.* 1986;40:97) • Sustained release formulations may bypass site of absorption
Ferrous sulfate 325 mg (65 mg elemental) 220 mg/5 mL (44 mg/5 mL elemental) 300 mg/mL (60 mg/5 mL elemental)		• Hemoglobin will rise slowly, generally 2 g/L over 2–3 weeks • A trial of IV iron or 1–3 months of PO iron can be considered for any CKD patient with TSAT ≤30% and ferritin ≤500 ng/mL (*Kidney Int Suppl.* 2012;2:279.)
Parenteral Iron[a]		
Ferumoxytol (Feraheme) 30 mg/mL (17 mL)	• CKD: 510 mg IV push every 3–8 days	• Common indications for IV iron therapy include ongoing blood loss, intolerance of or difficulty absorbing PO iron and cancer or dialysis patients taking ESAs who do not respond to or cannot take PO iron • Anaphylactic reactions have occurred with both iron dextran and sodium ferric gluconate, the reported frequency is 8.7 and 3.3 events per million, respectively (*Am J Kidney Dis.* 1999;33:464) • A 25 mg test dose is recommended by NCCN guidelines for sodium ferric gluconate in patients with history of anaphylaxis to iron dextran • Delayed (1–2 days) infusion reactions reported with iron dextran including arthralgias, dizziness, chills, and fever
Iron dextran (INFeD, Dexferrum) 50 mg/ml (1, 2 mL)	• Cancer: 25 mg test dose, followed 1 h later by 100 mg over 5 minutes • Labeled dosing = 0.0442 (desired Hgb – observed Hgb) × LBW + (0.26 × LBW)[b]	
Iron sucrose (Venofer) 20 mg/mL (5, 10 mL)	• CKD: 100–200 mg over 2–5 minutes 1–3 times per week up to 1 g cumulative dose • Cancer: 200 mg infused over 1 h every 2–3 weeks	
Sodium ferric gluconate (Ferrlecit) 12.5 mg/mL (5 mL)	• CKD: 125 mg over 1 h per dialysis session × 8 doses • Cancer: 125 mg over 1 h weekly × 8 doses	

[a]Parenteral iron product strengths reflect elemental iron content.
[b]LBW, lean body weight.

TABLE 11.1.2 Erythropoietin-Stimulating Agents for Treatment of Anemia

Drug	Indication	Dosing and Titration	Comments
Epoetin alfa (Epogen, Procrit)	CKD	Initial dose: • 50–100 units/kg 3 times/week Titration: • If Hgb ↑ >1 g/dL in 2 weeks, ↓ dose ≥25% • If Hgb <10 g/dL and does not ↑ by 1 g/dL after 4 weeks, ↑ dose 25% • Dialysis: If Hgb ≡ 11 g/dL ↓ dose or discontinue • Nondialysis: If Hgb ≡ 10 g/dL ↓ dose or discontinue	• Adverse effects include Hypertension (5–24%), thrombotic events, edema, fever, dizziness, insomnia, headache, pruritus, rash, nausea, constipation, vomiting, diarrhea, dyspepsia, injection site reactions, arthralgias, cough, seizure • Hgb response 2–6 weeks • Discontinue if response inadequate at 8 weeks (chemo) or 12 weeks (CKD) with appropriate doses • Evaluate BP, seizure, and VTE risk prior to initiating therapy • Epogen and Procrit contain human albumin
	Cancer	Initial dose: • 150 units/kg 3 times/week or 40,000 units/week Titration: • If Hgb ↑ >1 g/dL in 2 weeks, ↓ dose ≥25% • If Hgb <10 g/dL and does not ↑ by 1 g/dL after 2 weeks, ↑ dose 25%	

| Darbepoetin alfa (Aranesp) | CKD | Initial dose:
• Dialysis: 0.45 µg/kg/week, or 0.75 µg/kg/2 weeks
• Nondialysis: 0.45 µg/kg/4 weeks

Titration:
• If Hgb ↑ >1 g/dL in 2 weeks, ↓ dose 25%; if Hgb continues to increase, discontinue and resume when needed at ↓ dose
• If Hgb <10 g/dL and does not ↑ by 1g/dL after 4 weeks, ↑ dose 25%
• Dialysis: If Hgb ≅11 g/dL ↓ dose or discontinue
• Nondialysis: If Hgb ≅10 g/dL ↓ dose or discontinue | • Adverse effects include edema (21%), hypertension (4–20%), hypotension (20%), fatigue, fever, headache, dizziness, diarrhea, constipation, vomiting, nausea, muscle spasm, arthralgia, upper respiratory infection
• Aranesp available in albumin-containing and albumin-free
• IV dosing recommended for dialysis patients
• Aranesp SingleJect contains latex packaging
• Discontinue if response inadequate at 8 weeks (chemo) or 12 weeks (CKD) with appropriate doses
• Evaluate blood pressure, seizure, and VTE risk prior to initiating therapy |
| | Cancer | Initial dose:
• 2.25 µg/kg/week or 500 µg/3 weeks until completion of chemo

Titration:
• If Hgb <10 g/dL and does not ↑ by 1 g/dL after 6 weeks, ↑ dose to 4.5 µg/kg/week (weekly dosing; do not adjust if Q3 week dosing)
• If Hgb ↑ >1 g/dL in 2 weeks, or if sufficient to avoid RBC transfusion, ↓ dose 40%, if Hgb exceeds concentration needed to avoid transfusion, hold, and resume at 40% ↓ dose | |

Reproduced with permission from Ryan L. Anemia. In: Attridge R, Miller M, Moote R, Ryan L, eds. *Internal Medicine: A Guide to Clinical Therapeutics.* New York, NY: McGraw-Hill; 2012:chap 21.

TABLE 11.2.1 Risk Stratification and Indications for VTE Prophylaxis in Medical Inpatients

Category	VTE Risk (Padua Prediction Score)	VTE Risk (IMPROVE Risk Score)	Hemorrhagic Risk (IMPROVE Bleeding Risk)
Strongest risk factors	• Active cancer (3 pts) • Prior VTE (3 pts) • Reduced mobility (bed rest for at least 3 days—3 pts) • Known thrombophilia (3 pts)	• Previous VTE (3 pts) • Known thrombophilia (3 pts)	• Active gastroduodenal ulcer • Bleeding w/in 3 months prior to admission • Platelet count $<50,000/mm^3$
Other risk factors	• Trauma and/or surgery within past 1 month (2 pts) • Age ≥70 years old (1 pt) • Heart or respiratory failure (1 pt) • Acute MI or ischemic stroke (1 pt) • Acute infection or rheumatologic disease (1 pt) • BMI ≥30 (1 pt) • Ongoing hormonal therapy (1 pt)	• Cancer (1 pt) • Age >60 years old (1 pt)	• Increased age (≥85 vs. <40) • Hepatic failure (INR >1.5) • Severe renal failure (GFR <30 mL/min) • ICU or CCU admission • Central venous catheter • Rheumatic disease • Current cancer • Male sex
Score calculation	• Add points for each risk factor • ≥4 points is considered high risk (11% VTE risk)	• Calculate risk score at http://www.outcomes-umassmed.org/IMPROVE	
Prophylaxis indications	• No risk score has been prospectively and independently validated; use clinical judgement in determining use of prophylaxis • Consider pharmacologic prophylaxis for medical inpatients with high VTE risk (including critically ill patients) and low bleeding risk • Consider mechanical prophylaxis for medical inpatients with high VTE risk and high bleeding risk • See reference no. 4 for an in depth discussion of the risks, benefits, and indications for VTE prophylaxis		

Sources: (1) Barbar S, Noventa F, Rossetto V, et al. A risk assessment model for the identification of hospitalized medical patients at risk for venous thromboembolism: the Padua Prediction Score. *J Thromb Haemost.* 2010;8:2450–2457. (2) Spyropoulos AC, Anderson FA, Fitzgerald G, et al. Predictive and associative models to identify hospitalized patients at risk for VTE. *Chest.* 2011;140:706–714. (3) Decousus H, Tapson VF, Bergmann JF, et al. IMPROVE investigators. Factors at admission associated with bleeding risk in medical inpatients. *Chest.* 2011;139:69–79. (4) Kahn SR, Lim W, Dunn AS, et al. Prevention of VTE in non-surgical patients: antithrombotic therapy and prevention of thrombosis, 9th ed: American College of Chest Physicians Evidence-Based Clinical Practice Guidelines. *Chest.* 2012;141(2)(Suppl):195s–226s.

TABLE 11.2.2 Pharmacotherapy for VTE Prophylaxis

Drug	Indication	Dose	Comments
Parenteral Anticoagulants			
Unfractionated heparin	All indications	5000 U SC Q 8–12 h	• Enoxaparin 30–60 mg SC BID has been studied in bariatric surgery patients, it is unclear if these doses are beneficial in obese medical inpatients
Enoxaparin (Lovenox)	General medical or critically ill patients	40 mg SC Q 24 h	
	Hip replacement surgery	40 mg SC Q 24 h	• Dalteparin half-life prolonged if CrCl <30, no dose adjustment
		30 mg SC Q 12 h	provided by manufacturer, no significant accumulation with 5000
	Knee replacement surgery	30 mg SC Q 12 h	U SC daily dose for 7 days in patients with CrCl <30 (*Arch Int Med.*
	Abdominal surgery	40 mg SC Q 24 h	2008;168:1805)
	CrCl ≤30 mL/min	30 mg SC Q 24 h	• For dalteparin is contraindicated in patients weighing ≤50 kg or with CrCl <30 mL/min
Dalteparin (Fragmin)	General medical or critically ill patients	5000 U SC Q 24 h	• ACCP guidelines recommend prophylaxis for orthopedic procedures be initiated ≥12 h prior to or after surgery and continued for 10–14 days (*Chest.* 2012;141(2)(Suppl):e278)
	Hip replacement surgery	2500 U SC × 1 after surgery, then 5000 U SC Q 24 h	• ACCP guidelines recommend pharmacologic prophylaxis in abdominal surgery only in patients at moderate to high VTE risk and low bleeding
	Abdominal surgery	5000 U SC the evening prior to surgery then 5000 U SC Q 24 h	risk (*Chest.* 2012;141(2)(Suppl):e227)
Fondaparinux (Arixtra)	Medical inpatients, general and orthopedic surgery	2.5 mg Q 24 h	
Oral Anticoagulants			
Dabigatran (Pradaxa)	Hip or knee replacement surgery	110 mg PO 1–4 h post-surgery then 220 mg PO Q 24 h thereafter	• ACCP guidelines recommend LMWH over any other agent in orthopedic surgery (*Chest.* 2012;141(2)(Suppl):e278) • Dabigatran dosing reflects approved labelling in Canada, as of press time. Dabigatran was not approved in the United States for this
Rivaroxaban (Xarelto)	Hip or knee replacement surgery	10 mg Q 24 h	indication and the 110 mg strength was not available • Rivaroxaban not recommended for CrCl <30 mL/min
Warfarin	Hip or knee replacement surgery	Dose adjusted to INR 2–3	• Epidural catheters should not be pulled prior to 18 hours after the last dose of rivaroxaban, wait 6 hours to give subsequent dose.

TABLE 11.2.3 Pharmacotherapy for VTE Treatment

Drug	Dose	Comments
Parenteral Anticoagulants		
Dalteparin (Fragmin)	CrCl ≥20 mL/min 200 U/kg SC Q 24 h CrCl <30 mL/min Monitor anti-Xa levels	• Dalteparin max dose per manufacturer is 18000 U; dose response proven linear up to 190 kg with dalteparin and 144 kg for enoxaparin; experts recommend against dose capping in obese patients (*Ann Pharmacother.* 2009;43:1064.)
Enoxaparin (Lovenox)	CrCl >30 mL/min 1 mg/kg SC Q 12 h 1.5 mg/kg SC Q 24 h CrCl ≤30 mL/min 1 mg/kg SC Q 24 h	• Dalteparin is renally eliminated; no specific dose recommendations exist for renal impairment; the manufacturer recommends anti-Xa monitoring in patients with CrCl <30. • Higher recurrent VTE rates were observed in patients with BMI >27 taking enoxaparin 1.5 mg/kg Q 24 h (*Ann Int Med.* 2001;134:191.)
Fondaparinux (Arixtra)	<50 kg 5 mg SC Q 24 h 50–100 kg 7.5 mg SC Q 24 h >100 kg 10 mg SC Q 24 h CrCl 30–50 mL/min Reduce dose 50% CrCl <30 Contraindicated	• ACCP guidelines recommend either LMWH or fondaparinux over unfractionated heparin for VTE treatment (*Chest.* 2012 141(2)(Suppl):e419s) • Unfractionated heparin is not renally eliminated; consider for patients with CrCl ≤20 mL/min
Unfractionated heparin	80 U/kg bolus, then 18 U/kg/h IV infusion, titrate dose to target aPTT or heparin blood level 333 U/kg SC, followed by 250 U/kg SC Q 12 h (no monitoring required)	
Oral Anticoagulants		
Rivaroxaban (Xarelto)	15 mg PO Q 12 h for 3 weeks, then 20 mg PO Q 24 h	
Warfarin	Initiate 5 mg PO Q 24 h, titrate dose to INR 2–3 Alternatively, may initiate 10 mg PO Q 24 h times 2, then 5 mg PO Q 24 h	• Warfarin may be initiated at the same time as parenteral anticoagulants • Avoid the 10 mg × 2 starting dose in patients with risk of bleeding or hypercoagulable states • Consider initiating 2.5 mg PO Q 24 h in elderly patients

TABLE 11.2.4 Monitoring Anticoagulants for VTE Prophylaxis and Treatment

Drug	Indication	Assay	Target Range	Comments
Dalteparin (Fragmin)	VTE prophylaxis	Anti-Xa assay	0.2–0.5 IU/mL (5000 U dose)	• Draw assay 4 h after the 2nd or 3rd dose
	VTE treatment	Anti-Xa assay	1.05 IU/mL	
Enoxaparin (Lovenox)	VTE prophylaxis	Anti-Xa assay	0.2–0.4 IU/mL	**Adjustment nomogram** *(for 0.6–1.0 target)*:
	VTE treatment	Anti-Xa assay	0.6–1.0 IU/mL (1 mg/kg BID dose)	• Draw level 4 h after the 2nd or 3rd dose
				• <0.35 = ↑ dose 25%
			1.0–2.0 IU/mL (1.5 mg/kg QD dose)	• 0.35–0.49 = ↑ dose 10%
				• 0.5–1 = no change, redraw next day then weekly
				• 1.1–1.5 = ↓ dose 20%
				• 1.6–2 = hold × 3 h ↓ dose 30%
				• >2 = hold until <0.5 ↓ dose 40%
				• Redraw after next dose if not at target
Unfractionated heparin	VTE treatment	aPTT	1.5–2.5 times control value	**Adjustment nomogram** *(for heparin level 0.3–0.7 target)*:
		Heparin level (protamine titration assay)	0.2–0.4 U/mL	• Draw 6 h after bolus
				• <0.15 = 80 units/kg bolus and ↑ 4 units/kg/h
		Heparin level (antifactor Xa assay)	0.3–0.7 U/mL	• 0.15–0.29 = 40 units/kg bolus and ↑ 2 units/kg/h
				• 0.3–0.7 = no change
				• 0.71–1 = ↓ by 2 units/kg/h
				• >1 = hold × 1 h and ↓ 3 units/kg/h

(Continued)

TABLE 11.2.4 Monitoring Anticoagulants for VTE Prophylaxis and Treatment *(Continued)*

Drug	Indication	Assay	Target Range	Comments
Warfarin	VTE prophylaxis or treatment	INR	2–3	• Most patients with VTE should be treated for 3 months • Consider longer term therapy for patients with VTE secondary to cancer or with an unprovoked VTE at low risk of bleeding
	Recurrent VTE with APA syndrome	INR	2.5–3.5	• See reference no. 3 for full recommendations

Sources: (1) Nutescu EA, Spinler SA, Wittkowski A, Dager WE. Low-molecular-weight heparins in renal impairment and obesity: available evidence and clinical practice recommendations across medical and surgical settings. *Ann Pharmacother.* 2009;43:1064–1083. (2) Garcia DA, Baglin TP, Weitz JI, Samama MM. Parenteral anticoagulants: antithrombotic therapy and prevention of thrombosis, 9th ed: American College of Chest Physicians Evidence-Based Clinical Practice Guidelines. *Chest.* 2012;141(2)(Suppl):e24S–e43S. (3) Kearon C, Akl E, Comerota AJ, et al. Antithrombotic therapy for VTE disease: antithrombotic therapy and prevention of thrombosis, 9th ed: American College of Chest Physicians Evidence-Based Clinical Practice Guidelines. *Chest.* 2012;141(2)(Suppl):e419S–e494S.

TABLE 11.2.5 Selected Warfarin Drug Interactions

Interacting Drug	INR	Typical Onset	Clinical Implications
Amiodarone	↑	1–3 months	Potent 3A4 inibitor, high incidence of interaction
Valproic acid	↑	<24 h	Transient effect, no warfarin dose adjustment needed
Simvastatin, lovastatin, fluvastatin, rosuvastatin	↑	Within 1 week, potentially later	Simvastatin increased the INR 27% in one study (*Thromb Haemost.* 2003;89:949) consider atorvastatin or pravastatin
Phenobarbital	→	Between 1 week and 1 month	Decreases warfarin levels 38–40%
Fenofibrate	↑	Within 1 week	Supported by multiple case reports; consider empiric 20% reduction in warfarin dose (*Ann Pharmacother.* 2003;37:212); interaction is possible but appears less likely with gemfibrozil
Trimethoprim/Sulfamethoxazole	↑	2 days to 1 week	Supported by multiple case reports; consider empiric dose decrease or alternative antibiotic
Oxandrolone (and other anabolic steroids)	↑	Progressive over 4 weeks of initiation	In one study, the half-life of warfarin was doubled; monitor INR weekly until steady state
Duloxetine, fluoxetine	↑	1–2 months	In one case report, duloxetine caused an INR of 19 that fell once duloxetine was discontinued; consider citalopram, sertraline, paroxetine, escitalopram, venlafaxine, or cesvenlafaxine
Aprepitant	→	Within 3 days	A standard 3-day course of aprepitant causes an average INR decrease of 14%
Fluconazole, voriconazole, miconazole	↑	Poorly defined, likely within a few days	Interaction reported with miconazole oral and vaginal; itraconazole, ketoconazole, terbinafine, and posaconazole have lower chance of interaction

TABLE 11.3.1 Management of Excess Anticoagulation

Clinical Situation	Recommended Management
INR >5.0	If no significant bleed, omit or decrease dose
INR 5.0–9.0	If no significant bleed, omit 1–2 doses, hold warfarin, and give vitamin K 2.5 mg PO × 1
INR >9.0	If no significant bleeding, hold warfarin and give vitamin K 2.5–5 mg PO × 1
Serious bleeding on warfarin	Hold warfarin, give vitamin K 10 mg IV (administer over at least 10 minutes) plus FFP or PCC
Serious bleeding on unfractionated heparin drip	Stop heparin drip, administer protamine sulfate, 1 mg per 100 U heparin administered within the past 3 h
Serious bleeding while on subcutaneous unfractionated heparin	Hold heparin, administer protamine sulfate 1 mg per 100 U heparin dosed, give first 50 mg IV push over 10 minutes, infuse the remainder over 8–12 h
Serious bleeding while on subcutaneous enoxaparin	Hold enoxaparin, administer protamine sulfate 1 mg per 1 mg enoxaparin administered; may repeat 0.5 mg protamine per 1 mg enoxaparin if bleeding continues
Serious bleeding while on subcutaneous dalteparin	Hold dalteparin, administer protamine sulfate 1 mg per 100 U dalteparin administered; may repeat 0.5 mg protamine per 100 U dalteparin if bleeding continues

Sources: (1) Garcia DA, Baglin TP, Weitz JI, Samama MM. Parenteral anticoagulants: Antithrombotic therapy and prevention of thrombosis, 9th ed: American College of Chest Physicians Evidence-Based Clinical Practice Guidelines. Chest. 2012;141(2)(Suppl):e24S–e43S. (2) Ansell J, Hirsh J, Hylek E, et al. Pharmacology and management of the vitamin K antagonists, 8th ed: American College of Chest Physicians Evidence-Based Clinical Practice Guidelines. Chest 2008;133:160–198. (3) Ryan L. Anticoagulation. In: Atridge R, Miller M, Moote R, Ryan L, eds. Internal Medicine: A Guide to Clinical Therapeutics. New York, NY: McGraw-Hill; 2012.

TABLE 11.3.2 Pharmacotherapy for HIT

Drug	Dose	Comments
Argatroban	• Initial infusion 2 mcg/kg/min (actual body weight) • Lower initial infusion to 0.5–1.2 mcg/kg/min in heart failure, anasarca, critically ill patients with multiorgan dysfunction or postcardiac surgery • Measure aPTT 2 h after initiation, then maintain aPTT 1.5–3 times baseline • Transition to warfarin alone once INR on argatroban ≤2 mcg/kg/min and warfarin combined >4.0 • If argatroban dose >2 mcg/kg/min, reduce dose to 2 mcg/kg/min and measure INR 4–6 h post-dose reduction	*4Ts Pre-test probability for HIT:* • Thrombocytopenia: Platelet count fall: >50% and nadir >20,000 = 2 points; 30–50% or nadir 10–19,000 = 1 points; <30% or nadir <10,000 = 0 points • Timing of platelet count fall: Clear onset between days 5 and 10 or platelet count fall at ≤1 day if prior heparin exposure within the last 30 days = 2 points; consistent with fall at 5–10 days but unclear (e.g., missing platelet counts), onset after day 10, or fall ≤1 day with prior heparin exposure within 30–100 days = 1 point; platelet count fall at <4 days without recent exposure = 0 points • Thrombosis or other sequelae: Confirmed new thrombosis, skin necrosis, or acute systemic reaction after intravenous unfractionated heparin bolus = 2 points; progressive or recurrent thrombosis, nonnecrotizing (erythematous) skin lesions, or suspected thrombosis that has not been proven = 1 point; none = 0 points • Other causes for thrombocytopenia present: None apparent = 2 points; possible = 1 point; definite = 0 points • 4Ts interpretation Add points for each of the four above categories, resulting in a total score from 0 to 8. Pretest probabilities for HIT are 0–3 = low probability (0.9%); 4–5 = intermediate probability (11.4%); 6–8 = high probability (34%) • The washed platelet serotonin release assay and heparin-induced platelet activation assay are the most sensitive and specific for HIT • HIT antibody ELISA assays that detect only HIT IgG are more specific than assays that also detect other immunoglobulins • Argatroban is the treatment of choice in renal failure; lower doses required in advanced hepatic disease though specific dose recommendations are lacking • Initiate warfarin once platelets >150,000/mm³; overlap DTI until INR therapeutic
Bivalirudin (Angiomax)	• Initial infusion 0.15 mg/kg/h (normal renal function) • CrCl 30–60 mL/min: initial infusion 0.08–0.1 mg/kg/h • CrCl <30 mL/min: initial infusion 0.04–0.05 mg/kg/h • Target aPTT 1.5–2.5 times baseline	
Lepirudin (Refludan)	• IV bolus 0.2 mg/kg (bolus only indicated if thrombosis present) • Infusion: Initial 0.05–0.1 mg/kg/h; aPTT 4 h after initiation, then QD; maintain aPTT 1.5–2.5 times baseline • Titration: aPTT low = ↑ dose 20%; aPTT high = hold infusion for 1 h, then ↓ dose 50% • Maintain aPTT at 1.5 times baseline when starting warfarin and until warfarin INR 2–3; INR will decline slightly when lepirudin is withdrawn	

Sources: (1) Lo GK, Juhl D, Warkentin TE, et al. Evaluation of pretest clinical score (4 T's) for the diagnosis of heparin-induced thrombocytopenia in two clinical settings. *J Thromb Haemost.* 2006;4:759–765. (2) Linkins LA, Dans AL, Moores LK, et al. Treatment and prevention of heparin-induced thrombocytopenia: Antithrombotic Therapy and Prevention of Thrombosis, 9th ed: American College of Chest Physicians Evidence-Based Clinical Practice Guidelines. *Chest.* 2012;141:e495S–530S.

ABBREVIATIONS

ACS	Acute coronary syndrome	PEA	Pulseless electrical activity
ACLS	Advanced cardiovascular life support	RASS	Richmond agitation sedation scale
CI	Cardiac index	RSI	Rapid sequence intubation
CVD	Cardiovascular disease	SBP	Systolic blood pressure
CVP	Central venous pressure	$ScvO_2$	Central venous oxygen saturation
HR	Heart rate	SvO_2	Venous oxygen saturation
ICP	Intracranial pressure	VF	Ventricular fibrillation
IO	Intraosseous	VT	Ventricular tachycardia
MAP	Mean arterial pressure		

TABLE 12.1 Rapid Sequence Intubation

Agent	Dose	Indication	Comments
Pretreatment (not routinely indicated)			
Lidocaine	100 mg	Elevated ICP	Protects from elevated ICP
Fentanyl	2–3 µg/kg	Elevated ICP, CVD	Decreases catecholamine surge
Induction			
Etomidate	0.3 mg/kg	Emergency RSI	May cause adrenal insufficiency
Ketamine	1.5 mg/kg	RSI in patients septic or with reactive airways	Caution in CVD and in hypertensive patients. May pretreat with atropine
Propofol	1.5 mg/kg	RSI with reactive airway or status epilepticus	Negative effects on CV system; bolus dosing may cause hypotension
Midazolam	0.2–0.3 mg/kg	Alternative for RSI	Variable response
Paralytic			
Succinylcholine	1.5 mg/kg	Agent of choice for RSI	Avoid in patients with hyperkalemia
Rocuronium	1 mg/kg	RSI when succinylcholine contraindicated	Duration up to 60 min; activity prolonged in patients with hepatic failure
Vecuronium	0.15 mg/kg	Used when succinylcholine and rocuronium not available	Duration up to 60 min; priming dose of 0.01 mg/kg give prior to RSI dose; activity prolonged in patients with renal and hepatic failure

TABLE 12.2.1 Sedation Agents

Agent	Starting Dose	Titration[a]	Comments
Propofol	5–20 µg/ kg/min	5 µg/kg/min Q 5 min	Max rate 50 µg/kg/min (institutional dependant); adverse effects: hypotension, high lipid content (1.1 kcal/mL), myocardial depressant. Sulfites in some formulations
Midazolam	1 mg/h	1 mg/h Q 15 min	CYP 3A4 interactions; benzyl alcohol in injection
Lorazepam	0.5 mg/h	0.5–1 mg/h Q 15 min	Propylene glycol and polyethylene glycol in injection. Reduce dose by 50% with concomitant valproic acid use. Use caution with renal and hepatic impairment
Dexmedetomidine	0.4 µg/kg/h	0.1 µg/kg/h Q 15 min	Max rate 0.7 µg/kg/h; dose-related bradycardia and hypotension; add adjunctive midazolam. FDA indicated for 24-h use; data available for 5-day use

[a]Titration should be based on RASS.

TABLE 12.2.2 Opioid Agents

Agent	Starting Dose	Titration[a]	Comments
Morphine	1 mg/h	1 mg/h Q 1 h	Prolonged activity in renal failure, hypotension, bronchospasm
Hydromorphone	0.2 mg/h	0.2 mg/h Q 1 h	Prolonged activity in renal and hepatic failure, hypotension
Fentanyl	25 µg/h	25–50 µg/h Q 15 min	Not prolonged in renal failure, chest wall rigidity with high-dose infusions

[a]Titration should be based on RASS and Pain Scale.

TABLE 12.2.3 Paralytic Agents

Agent	Bolus Dose	Infusion Starting Dose	Maximum Dose	Comments
Cisatracurium	0.1 mg/kg	2 µg/kg/min	10 µg/kg/min	No activity prolongation in renal or hepatic failure
Vecuronium	0.1 mg/kg	0.8 µg/kg/min	1.7 µg/kg/min	Prolonged activity in renal failure and hepatic failure
Rocuronium	0.6 mg/kg	4 µg/kg/min	16 µg/kg/min	Prolonged activity in hepatic failure

Pearls

- Monitoring should be through the Train of Four (TOF). This measures peripheral nerve stimulation using four electrical impulses
- Titration should be to a goal of TOF: 2/4
- Agents that increase potential blockade include corticosteroids, aminoglycosides, clindamycin, tetracyclines, colistin, calcium channel blockers, furosemide, lithium, and type 1 a antiarrhythmics

TABLE 12.3 Vasopressors and Inotropes

Agent	Dose (Goal)	Titration (Max Dose)	Comments
Vasopressors			
Dopamine	2.5 µg/kg/min (MAP >60)	2.5 µg/kg/min Q 5 min (20 µg/kg/min)	1–3 µg/kg/min = dopaminergic; 3–10 µg/kg/min = beta-1 stimulation; >10 µg/kg/min = alpha 1 vasoconstriction; not compatible with bicarbonate
Norepinephrine	5–10 µg/min OR 0.1 µg/kg/min (MAP >60)	10 µg/min Q 5 min (30 µg/min)	Primarily increases systemic vascular resistance; if extravasation occurs, treat with phentolamine IV 5–10 mg; not compatible with bicarbonate
Epinephrine	1 µg/min OR 0.1 µg/kg/min (MAP >60; CI >2)	1 µg/min Q 5 min (10 µg/min)	Positive inotropic and chronotropic effects; not compatible with bicarbonate
Phenylophrine	25 µg/min OR 0.5 µg/kg/min (MAP >60)	25 µg/min Q 5 min (180 µg/min)	Pure alpha agonist with minimal cardiac effect; compatible with bicarbonate
Vasopressin	0.04 units/min	Fixed dose (0.04 units/min)	Beneficial during acidosis and hypoxia; Y-site compatible with bicarbonate
Inotropes			
Dobutamine	2.5 µg/kg/min (MAP >60; CI > 2)	2.5 µg/kg/min Q 5 min	Increases cardiac output; may cause hypotension due to beta stimulation. Do not administer in same line with heparin, hydrocortisone, cefazolin, and penicillin; not compatible with bicarbonate
Milrinone	0.25 µg/kg/min (MAP >60; CI > 2)	0.25 µg/kg/min Q 10 min (0.75 µg/kg/min)	Adjust dose for renal failure; Y-site and syringe compatible with bicarbonate

TABLE 12.4 Intravenous Antihypertensives[a]

Agent	Dose	Titration	Comments
Diltiazem	5 mg/h	5 mg/h Q 15 min	Utilized in atrial fibrillation cases; not routinely used for hypertensive emergencies; max 15 mg/h
Esmolol	50 µg/kg/min	50 µg/kg/min Q 5–10 min	Preferred in aortic dissection; max rate 300 µg/kg/min
Labetalol	0.5 mg/min	0.5 mg/min Q 5 min	Preferred in acute stroke; max 300 mg/24 h
Nicardipine	5 mg/h	5 mg/h Q 15 min	Preferred in acute stroke; max 15 mg/h; may cause reflex tachycardia; caution with coronary ischemia
Nitroglycerin	5 µg/min	5 µg/min Q 3–5 min	Preferred in ACS; max rate of 100 µg/min
Nitroprusside	0.5 µg/kg/min	0.5 µg/kg/min Q 3–5 min	Preferred in acute heart failure; max rate 3 µg/kg/min; cyanide toxicity; caution in renal and hepatic disease; caution with elevated ICP
Clevidipine	1 mg/h	1 mg/h Q 5–10 min	Max rate of 32 mg/h; formulation contains egg and soy products; caution in patients with lipid disorders
Hydralazine	5–10 mg Q 4–6 h	No drip	Preferred in eclampsia; reflex tachycardia
Enalaprilat	0.625 mg Q 4–6 h	No drip	Max of 5 mg Q 6 h; avoid in acute renal failure
Phentolamine	5–20 mg Q 2–4 h	No drip	Used for adrenergic crises

[a]See Table 1.1.7 for treatment of hypertensive emergencies.

TABLE 12.5 Drugs for Atrial Fibrillation with Rapid Ventricular Response

Agent	Loading Dose	Maintenance Dose	Titration (Goal)	Comments
Diltiazem	0.25 mg/kg	5–15 mg/h	5 mg/h Q 15 min (SBP <160; HR <100)	Avoid in systolic heart failure
Verapamil	0.075–0.15 mg/kg	No infusion	N/A	Avoid in systolic heart failure
Esmolol	500 µg/kg	50–200 µg/kg/min	50 µg/kg/min Q 5–10 min (SBP <160; HR <100)	Avoid in asthmatics
Metoprolol	2.5–5 mg	No infusion	N/A	Give for 3 doses; caution in asthmatics
Propranolol	0.15 mg/kg	No infusion	N/A	Avoid in asthmatics
Amiodarone	150 mg	0.5–1 mg/min	Fixed	Several toxicities: pulmonary, skin, thyroid, optic, hepatic; can be used in patients with an accessory pathway
Digoxin	0.5 mg × 1, then 0.25 mg Q 6 h × 2 doses; OR 0.25 Q 2 h, up to 1.5 mg	0.125–0.25 mg/day	N/A (HR <100)	Check digoxin level (0.8–2.0 ng/mL); reduce maintenance dose in renal insufficiency

TABLE 12.6.1 Cardiac Arrest

Agent	Indication	Dose	Comments
Epinephrine	VF/pulseless VT/asystole/PEA	1 mg IV Q 3–5 min	1 mg IO can be utilized if no IV; 2–2.5 mg endotracheally can also be given
Vasopressin	VF/pulseless VT/asystole/PEA	40 units IV	Can replace 1st or 2nd epinephrine dose; can also be given IO
Amiodarone	VF/pulseless VT	300 mg	Can repeat with 150 mg
Lidocaine	VF/pulseless VT	1–1.5 mg/kg	Follow with 0.5–0.75 mg/kg Q 5–10 min (max 3 mg/kg); utilized if amiodarone not available
Magnesium	VF/pulseless VT with torsades de pointes	1–2 g in 10 mL of D5W	Routine administration not recommended unless torsades de pointes present
Sodium bicarbonate	Acidosis, tricyclic overdose	1 mEq/kg	Not standard in codes, utilized in specific scenarios

TABLE 12.6.2 Supraventricular Tachyarrhythmia

Agent	Dose	Comments
Adenosine	6 mg	Repeat with 12 mg; caution with bronchospasm; interacts with carbamazepine, caffeine, theophylline
Diltiazem	0.25 mg/kg	Infuse at 5–15 mg/h; avoid in heart failure; use in narrow complex
Verapamil	2.5–5 mg	Repeat 5 mg Q 10 min; max = 30 mg
Metoprolol	5 mg	Repeat every 15 min to max 15 mg; avoid in pre-excited atrial fibrillation/atrial flutter
Esmolol	500 µg/kg	Infuse at 50 µg/kg/min; avoid in pre-excited atrial fibrillation/atrial flutter
Procainamide	100 mg	Give every 5 min until arrhythmia controlled or hypotension occurs, QRS prolongs by 50%, or cumulative dose of 17 mg/kg is met; use in pre-excited atrial fibrillation
Amiodarone	150 mg over 10 min	Infuse at 1 mg/min for 6 hr, then 0.5 mg/min [total dose over 24 h (should not exceed 2.2 g/24hr)]
Digoxin	0.5 mg × 1; then 0.25 mg Q 6 h × 2 doses	Maintenance of 0.125–0.25 mg/day; slow onset of action

TABLE 12.6.3 Ventricular Tachyarrhythmia

Agent	Indication	Dose	Comments
Amiodarone	Stable monomorphic VT; polymorphic VT with normal QT interval	150 mg over 10 min	Infuse at 1 mg/min for 6 hr, then 0.5 mg/min (total dose over 24 h)
Procainamide	Stable monomorphic VT	100 mg	Give every 5 min until arrhythmia controlled or hypotension occurs, QRS prolongs by 50%, or cumulative dose of 17 mg/kg is met
Sotalol	Stable monomorphic VT	1.5 mg/kg over 5 min	Avoid in QT prolongation and CHF
Lidocaine	Stable monomorphic VT	1–1.5 mg/kg	Follow with 0.5–0.75 mg/kg Q 5–10 min (max 3 mg/kg); follow with infusion of 1–4 mg/min
Magnesium	Polymorphic VT associated with torsades de pointes	1–2 g in 10 mL of D5W	Utilized if torsades is present

TABLE 12.6.4 Bradycardia

Agent	Dose	Comments
Atropine	0.5 mg IV	Give every 3–5 min (max 3 mg)
Dopamine	2–10 µg/kg/min	
Epinephrine	2–10 µg/kg/min	

TABLE 12.7 Sepsis Treatment Goals

Variable	Goal	Intervention	Comments
CVP	8–12	If <8, give normal saline bolus (500 mL) and aggressive fluid resuscitation (rate 150–200 mL/h)	Colloids can also be utilized
SBP/MAP	90–140 mm Hg/65–90	If <90 mm Hg/<65, initiate vasopressor therapy; evaluate adrenal glands (ACTH stimulation test)	ACTH stimulation test: Give ACTH 250 µg IV; measure cortisol at 0,30, and 60 min; give dexamethasone 2 mg IV Q 6 h while stimulation test results are pending
SvO_2 $ScvO_2$	≥65 ≥70	If $ScvO_2$ <70 and Hgb <10 g/dL, transfuse blood; If $ScvO_2$ <70 and Hgb >10 g/dL start dobutamine drip	Give dobutamine if HR <100 and SBP >100
HR	≤120	If >120, reevaluate vasopressors	
Lactate	<2	If >2, recheck in 4–6 h	
Infectious source	Source control	Surgical intervention as needed; broad spectrum antibiotics	Reassess antibiotics every 12–24 h based on culture and sensitivity

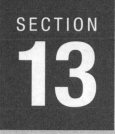

SECTION

13

Fluids and Electrolytes

ABBREVIATIONS

ADH	Antidiuretic hormone	NDI	Nephrogenic diabetes insipidus
CDI	Central diabetes insipidus	½ NS	Half-normal saline (0.45% saline)
D5W	Dextrose 5%	NS	Normal saline
DDAVP	Desmopressin	UOP	Urine output
DI	Diabetes insipidus	SIADH	Syndrome of inappropriate antidiuretic hormone
HCTZ	Hydrochlorothiazide		
LR	Lactated ringers		

TABLE 13.1.1.1 Fluid Composition and Uses

Fluid Composition	Main Indications	Comments	Dosing
Hypotonic Fluids			
D5W	Fluid maintenance	May impair glucose control in diabetes; provides free water to all compartments	• Maintenance dosing according to the 4:2:1 rule: • 4 mL/kg/hr for 1–10 kg • Add 2 mL/kg/h for 10–20 kg • Add 1 mL/kg/h for every kg over 20 kg
½ NS—0.45% NaCl (Na⁺ 77 mEq/L, Cl⁻ 77 mEq/L)	Fluid maintenance	Hyponatremia with long-term use; increased risk of IV infiltration vs. isotonic	
Isotonic Fluids			
NS—0.9% NaCl (Na⁺ 154 mEq/L, Cl⁻ 154 mEq/L)	Fluid replacement; hypovolemia, shock	Monitor for fluid overload; hyperchloremic metabolic acidosis with large volumes	• Dose varies widely depending on patient fluid status and clinical situation
LR (Na⁺ 130 mEq/L, Cl⁻ 109 mEq/L Lactate 28 mEq/L, K⁺ 4 mEq/L Ca⁺⁺ 3 mEq/L)	Fluid replacement; hypovolemia	Lactate converted to bicarbonate in the liver, may accumulate in cirrhosis leading to lactic acidosis	
Hypertonic Fluids			
3% NaCl (Na⁺ 513 mEq/L, Cl⁻ 513 mEq/L)	Severe symptomatic hyponatremia	Osmotic demyelination syndrome with too-rapid correction (>12 mEq/L/d for acute hyponatremia, >8 mEq/L/d for chronic hyponatremia)	• Initial rate = desired serum [Na⁺] increase per hour (mEq/h) × patient weight (kg) (example: ↑ Na⁺ by 1 mEq/L/h in 70 kg patient = 70 mL/h infusion, *Am J Med.* 2007;120(11A):S1) • Alternate calculation: Effect of 1 L 3% saline on serum [Na⁺] = (513 − serum Na⁺)/(TBW+1), where TBW = 0.6 × weight (kg) for males, 0.5 × weight (kg) for females, rate to raise 1 mEq/L/hr = 1/(Effect of 1 L 3% saline on serum [Na⁺])

FIGURE 13.1.2 Evaluation Algorithm for Hyponatremia

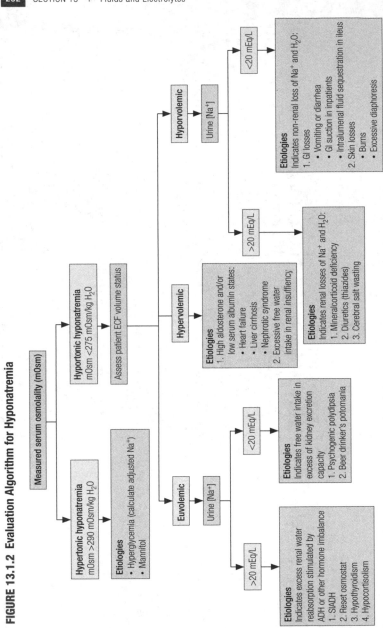

(Continued)

FIGURE 13.1.3 Treatment Algorithm for Hyponatremia

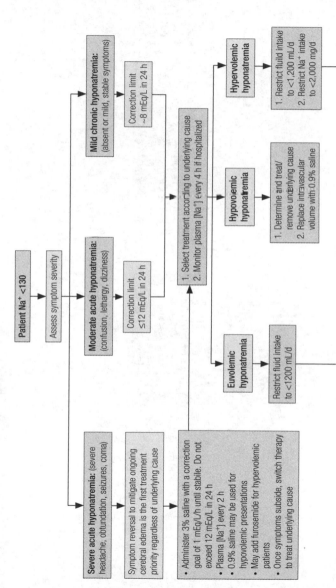

Patient Na⁺ <130

Assess symptom severity

Severe acute hyponatremia: (severe headache, obtundation, seizures, coma)

Symptom reversal to mitigate ongoing cerebral edema is the first treatment priority regardless of underlying cause

- Administer 3% saline with a correction goal of 1 mEq/L/h until stable. Do not exceed 12 mEq/L in 24 h
- Plasma [Na⁺] every 2 h
- 0.9% saline may be used for hypovolemic presentations
- May add furosemide for hypervolemic patients
- Once symptoms subside, switch therapy to treat underlying cause

Moderate acute hyponatremia: (confusion, lethargy, dizziness)

Correction limit ≤12 mEq/L in 24 h

Mild chronic hyponatremia: (absent or mild, stable symptoms)

Correction limit ~8 mEq/L in 24 h

1. Select treatment according to underlying cause
2. Monitor plasma [Na⁺] every 4 h if hospitalized

Euvolemic hyponatremia

Restrict fluid intake to <1200 mL/d

Hypovolemic hyponatremia

1. Determine and treat/remove underlying cause
2. Replace intravascular volume with 0.9% saline

Hypervolemic hyponatremia

1. Restrict fluid intake to <1,200 mL/d
2. Restrict Na⁺ intake to <2,000 mg/d

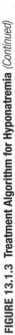

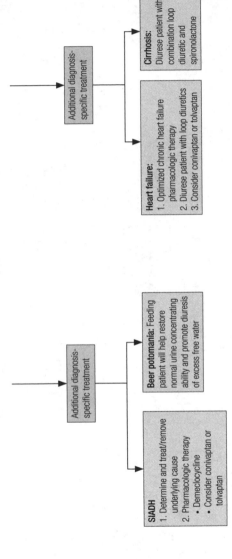

FIGURE 13.1.3 Treatment Algorithm for Hyponatremia (*Continued*)

Additional diagnosis-specific treatment

Heart failure:
1. Optimized chronic heart failure pharmacologic therapy
2. Diurese patient with loop diuretics
3. Consider conivaptan or tolvaptan

Cirrhosis: Diurese patient with combination loop diuretic and spironolactone

Additional diagnosis-specific treatment

SIADH
1. Determine and treat/remove underlying cause
2. Pharmacologic therapy
 • Demeclocycline
 • Consider conivaptan or tolvaptan

Beer potomania: Feeding patient will help restore normal urine concentrating ability and promote diuresis of excess free water

FIGURE 13.1.4 Assessment and Treatment Algorithm of Hypernatremia

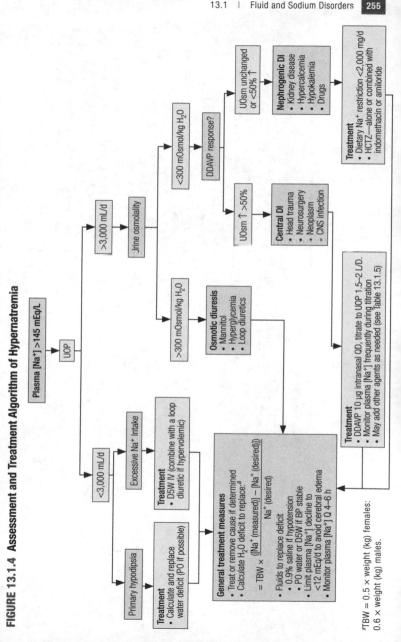

TABLE 13.1.5 Pharmacotherapy of Sodium Disorders

Drug	Indication	Dosing	Comments
Hyponatremia			
3% saline	Acute hyponatremia with severe symptoms	Infusion rate = desired [Na$^+$] ↑ per hour (mEq/h) × weight (kg) (see Table 13.1.1)	• Limit serum [Na$^+$] correction to ≤12 mEq/L/d for acute, ≤8 mEq/L/d for chronic hyponatremia to prevent osmotic demyelination • Total daily correction more predictive of osmotic demyelination than hourly correction rate (*Kidney Int.* 1992;41(6):1662)
Demeclocycline	Chronic, mild SIADH	Initiate 300 mg BID; max 600 mg BID; 3–4 days for max effect	• Dizziness, headache, nausea, and common diarrhea can be nephrotoxic • Take on empty stomach; do not take with dairy products or antacids due to deactivation from chelation • Avoid in renal dysfunction • Peak effect in 3–4 days
Conivaptan (Vaprisol)	Hypervolemic hyponatremia secondary to heart failure or acute symptomatic SIADH	Load 20 mg IV over 30 min, then 20 mg infused over 24 h; up to 4 days	• May cause hypotension or infusion site pain (use central line) • Limit serum [Na$^+$] correction to ≤12 mEq/L/d for acute, ≤8 mEq/L/d for chronic hyponatremia to prevent osmotic demyelination • Avoid in patients with cirrhosis due to potential for hypotension from V1 a receptor blockade (*Kidney Int.* 2006;69:2124)
Tolvaptan (Samsca)	Chronic SIADH, hypervolemic hyponatremia	Initiate 15 mg PO QD; max 60 mg PO QD	• Onset within 24 h • Dosing can be limited by thirst stimulation

Hypernatremia			
DDAVP	CDI along with fluid restriction	Intranasal: Initial 0.1 mg QD; max 0.2 mg BID SC: 0.1–0.2 mg BID PO: 0.1 mg QD	• 1st line for CDI • Titrate to UOP 1.5–2 L/d • More predictable response with intranasal than PO • SC and PO forms are approximately 1/10th the potency of intranasal with high inter-patient variability
HCTZ	NDi; CDI along with DDAVP	25 mg QD up to BID	• 1st line for NDI
Indomethacin	NDI along with HCTZ	50 mg Q8–12 h	• Counteracts renal prostaglandin inhibition of ADH
Amiloride	NDI along with HCTZ	5–10 mg QD	• 1st line for NDI secondary to Li$^+$ • Monitor for hyperkalemia • May combine with HCTZ

TABLE 13.2.1 Potassium and Magnesium Repletion

Replacement	Products	Dosing	Comments
Oral potassium chloride[a]	Tablets: 8, 10, 20 mEq XR Powder: 20 mEq	10–40 mEq PO up to 4 times daily	• K+ deficit estimate: 10 mEq per every 0.1 mEq serum K+ 3.0–3.5; 20 mEq per every 0.1 mEq serum K+ <3.0 • Use PO for mild or asymptomatic hypokalemia
IV potassium chloride[a]	KCl injection	Peripheral access: 10 mEq/h Central access: 10–20 mEq/h usual, up to 40 mEq/h in large volume	• IV for symptomatic or severe hypokalemia • Telemetry monitoring for IV rate >10 mEq/h • May use K-Phos if concomitant hypophosphatemia, see Table 13.3.1
Oral magnesium oxide	Tablets: 400 mg (Mag-Ox) Capsules: 140 mg (Uro-Mag)	400 mg with meals	• Hypokalemia is difficult to correct without correcting concurrent hypomagnesemia • Oral magnesium is better absorbed with food
Oral magnesium chloride	Tablet: 64 mg (Slow-Mag, Mag 64)	64–128 mg with meals	• Magnesium chloride tablets also contain ~110 mg Ca++ • Diarrhea common with magnesium oxide
Oral magnesium lactate	Tablet: 84 mg (Mag-Tab SR)	84–168 mg with meals	• 50% magnesium excreted in urine, may require several days of therapy for full repletion, in particular for oral route
IV magnesium sulfate	MgSO4 40 or 80 mg/mL infusion	1–2 g/h infusion, repeat as needed	

[a]Potassium also available as phosphate salt (K-Phos), see Table 13.3.1 for available preparations and dosing.

TABLE 13.2.2 Pharmacotherapy of Hyperkalemia

Drug	Dosing	Comments
Step 1—Cardioprotection		
Calcium gluconate: 10% 1 g; 10, 50, 100 mL vials	1 g IV push over 2 min; may repeat Q10 min	• 1 g = 93 mg elemental Ca^{++} • Effect is transient, repeat Q 10 min as needed
Step 2—Shift K$^+$ Intracellular		
Insulin (regular): 100 units/mL 10 mL vial	10 units IV; may infuse in 500 mL D5 W or bolus + 1 amp D50	• Decreased [K$^+$] 0.5 – 1.0 mEq/L (*Nephrol Dial Transplant.* 1989;4(3):228) • 20 min onset; duration 4–6 h
Albuterol: 2.5 mg/3 mL	10 mg nebulized	• Similar onset/efficacy as insulin; efficacy is additive • Hypoglycemia can occur when given with insulin (*Kidney Int.* 1990;38:869) • Tachycardia is common; may precipitate angina in CAD
Sodium bicarbonate: 50 mEq/50 mL vial	150 mEq in 1 L D5W; infuse over 4 h	• Use only in setting of metabolic acidosis; may repeat if needed; requires ≥4 h to take effect (*Kidney Int.* 1992;41:369)
Step 3—Remove K$^+$		
Sodium polystyrene sulfonate: 15 g/4 teaspoons powder	15 g PO or retention enema up to QID	• Forms with sorbitol not recommended secondary to risk of intestinal necrosis (*J Am Soc Nephrol.* 2010;21:733) • Onset ~1 h; duration ~6 h
Furosemide: 10 mg/mL vial	20–80 mg IV Q6 h	• Limited data on use; add NS infusion if volume depleted

TABLE 13.3.1 Calcium and Phosphorus Repletion

Drug	Dosage Forms	Dosing[a]	Comments
Oral Calcium			
Calcium carbonate	Tablets and suspension (many strengths)	1,000–2,000 mg per day elemental calcium[b] given with meals	• 40% elemental calcium • Acidic pH required for maximal absorption; take with food; absorption reduced by PPIs and H2 blockers
Calcium citrate	Tablets (many strengths)	1,000–2,000 mg elemental calcium[b] divided 2 to 3 times per day	• 21% elemental calcium • pH-independent absorption (may take with or without food)
IV Calcium			
Calcium chloride	100 mg/mL injection	1 g slow IV push (over 10 min) in a central line or 1–2 g in 100 mL (D5 W or NS) infused over 1 h, repeat as needed	• 27.3% elemental calcium • Requires central line secondary to vein irritation • Do not give IM or SC due to severe tissue injury • IV calcium reserved for symptomatic hypocalcemia
Calcium gluconate	500 mg tablet; 100 mg/mL injection	1 g IV push or 1–2 g in 100 mL (D5 W or NS) infused over 15 min, repeat as needed	• 9.3% elemental calcium • IV calcium reserved for symptomatic hypocalcemia • May infuse in peripheral vein or give IM

Oral Phosphate			
Potassium phosphate	Neutra-Phos-K (8 mmol PO_4/14.25 mEq K^+) granules	1–3 packets 3 times daily	• 8 mmol PO_4 = 250 mg PO_4 • Use low K^+ formulation if normal or high serum [K^+] (see sodium–potassium phosphate below)
Sodium–potassium phosphate	8 mmol PO_4 with varying amounts of Na^+ and K^+ (see comments)	1–3 packets/tablets 3 times daily	• Neutra-Phos (8 mmol PO_4/7 mEq Na^+/7 mEq K^+) granules • K-Phos Neural (8 mmol PO_4/13 mEq Na^+/1.1 mEq K^+) tablets • Uro-KP-Neutral (8 mmol PO_4/10.9 mEq Na^+/1.27 mEq K^+) tablets
IV Phosphate			
Sodium phosphate	3 mmol PO_4/4 mEq Na^+ per mL Injection	15 mmol PO_4 in 250 mL (D5W or ½NS) or 30 mmol in 250 mL D5W infused over 3 h, repeat as needed	• 15 mmol in 250 mL ½ NS or 30 mmol in 250 mL D5W produce an isotonic solution • Do not administer to patients with hypercalcemia or co-administer with IV calcium
Potassium phosphate	3 mmol PO_4/4.4 mEq K^+ per mL injection	15 mmol PO_4 (22 mEq K^+) in 250 mL (NS or D5W) infused over 3 h, repeat as needed	• May give 30 mmol over 3 h through central line • Do not administer to patients with hypercalcemia or coadminister with IV calcium • Mean serum [PO_4] increase 3 h post infusion = 0.80 mg/dL and 1.34 mg/dL with 15 mmol and 30 mmol dose respectively (*Ann Pharmacother.* 1997;31:683)

[a]Calcium dosing represents requirement for replacing calcium in hypocalcemic patients and does not reflect calcium supplementation dosing for other indications.
[b]Check the product label closely. Some calcium supplements have the elemental dosing on the label and some do not.

TABLE 13.3.2 Pharmacotherapy of Hypercalcemia

Drug	Dosing	Comments
Fluid Resuscitation		
0.9% saline; premixed bags	200 mL/h initially	• First-line therapy • Restores intravascular volume and improves renal Ca^{++} excretion • Titrate to maintain UOP 100–150 mL/h
Bisphosphonates		
Pamidronate (Aredia); 30, 90 mg vial	60–90 mg IV over 2–24 h	• Onset of activity is 48 h • ~25% of patients will experience flu-like illness within 3 days of administration; symptoms include fever, arthralgias, and myalgias • Can be nephrotoxic: safe level of renal impairment for use not clearly established; zoledronic acid studied in SCr up to 4.5 mg/dL; extend infusion time and ensure adequate hydration in renal insufficiency
Zoledronic acid (Zometa) 4 mg vial	4 mg IV over 15–60 min	
Ibandronate (Boniva); 3 mg vial	2–4 mg IV over 2 h	
Adjunct Treatments		
Calcitonin; 400 IU vial	4 IU/kg Q 12 h	• Onset within 6 h; efficacy limited to 48 h due to development of tolerance • Use with fluids and bisphosphonates safe to use in renal failure • Allergic reactions, incidence rare but may be severe
Glucocorticoids; numerous preparations	20–60 mg/d prednisone or equivalent	• Onset 2–5 days • Inhibit intestinal Ca^{++} absorption, therefore most effective in hypercalcemia from excess vitamin D (sarcoidosis, excess intake) • Gradually taper dose once serum [Ca^{++}] stable
Gallium nitrate; 25 mg/mL vial	200 mg/m^2; 24 h infusion up to 5 days	• 48 h onset • Nephrotoxicity 8–12.5% (Prod Info Ganite, 2003) • Contraindicated if SCr >2.5

ABBREVIATIONS			
AKI	Acute kidney injury	IR	Immediate release
COX	Cyclooxygenase	NSAID	Nonsteroidal anti-inflammatory drug
CR	Controlled release	TDS	Transdermal system
ER	Extended release	VAS	Visual analog scale
ICP	Intracranial pressure	XR	Extended release

TABLE 14.1.1 NSAID and Acetaminophen Dosing

Drug	Dosing	Comments
Nonselective NSAIDs (COX-1 and 2 inhibitors)		
Aspirin	325–1,000 mg PO Q 4–6 h	• Though data are limited, it appears other NSAIDs may interfere with the antiplatelet effects of aspirin (*J Clin Pharm.* 2008;48:117; *J Am Coll Cardiol.* 2004;43:985.); administer NSAIDs 2 h after aspirin
Diclofenac	50 mg PO Q 8 h	
Etodolac	200–400 mg PO Q 6–8 h	• IV ketorolac should be limited to 5 days of therapy due to risk of AKI (*Ann Int Med.* 1997;126:193)
Fenoprofen	200 mg PO Q 4–6 h	• NSAIDs are one of the most commonly implicated drugs leading to hospitalization due to an adverse effect (*Br J Clin Pharmacol.* 2007;63:136), see Table 14.1.2
Ibuprofen	200–400 mg PO Q 4–6 h	
Ketoprofen	25–50 mg PO Q 6–8 h	• In patients requiring an NSAID: consider naproxen if high CV risk, consider a COX-2 inhibitor if high GI risk; consider adding a PPI to naproxen if high CV and GI risk (*Aliment Pharmacol Ther.* 2009;29:481)
Ketorolac	15–30 mg IV Q 6 h	
Naproxen	250 mg PO Q 6–8 h, or 500 mg PO Q 12 h	
Selective NSAIDs (COX-2 inhibitors)		
Celecoxib	200 mg PO Q 12 h	• Meloxicam and nabumetone lose COX-2 selectivity at higher doses; more GI bleeds observed with 15 mg vs. 7.5 mg meloxicam (*Am J Med.* 2004;117:100)
Meloxicam	7.5–15 mg PO QD	
Nabumetone	1,000–2,000 mg PO QD	• Cross-sensitivity to celecoxib in sulfonamide allergic patients appears low (*Drug Safety.* 2003;26:187)
Other		
Acetaminophen	325–1,000 mg PO Q 4–6 h	• Historically, the maximum daily dose of acetaminophen has been 4 g/day (2 g in liver disease); in 2011 the FDA suggested lowering this limit to 2.6 g/day and to avoid acetaminophen in patients with liver disease over concerns for increasing incidence of overdose

TABLE 14.1.2 NSAID Adverse Effects

Organ System	Adverse Effects	Comments
Cardiovascular	• Heart failure exacerbation • Increased risk of MI in patients with CAD • Hypertension	• ACC/AHA recommends avoiding NSAIDs when possible in patients with heart failure (*Circulation.* 2009;119(14):e391) or post-MI (*J Am Coll Cardiol.* 2007;50:e1) • Naproxen appears to have lower risk of MI (*Aliment Pharmacol Ther.* 2009;29:481) • Increased hospitalizations for heart failure associated with NSAIDs (*Arch Intern Med.* 2009;169:141) likely secondary to fluid retention and systemic vasoconstriction • Short- and long-term NSAIDs are associated with slight increased risk of MI and death in patients with a history of MI (*Circulation.* 2011;123:2226); naproxen appears to have the lowest risk • Slight elevation in blood pressure and slightly diminished effectiveness of antihypertensives observed with NSAIDs (*Semin Nephrol.* 1995;14:244); effect appears low with aspirin (*Ann Int Med.* 1994;121:289)
Gastrointestinal	• Dyspepsia • Gastric and duodenal ulcers	Gastroduodenal toxicity risk per the American College of Gastroenterology (*Am J Gastroenterol.* 2009;104:728.): • High risk = H/o of complicated PUD, >2 moderate risk factors • Moderate risk = Age >65 years old, high-dose NSAIDs, h/o uncomplicated ulcer, concurrent aspirin, corticosteroid or anticoagulant use • Low risk = No risk factors
Hematologic	• Platelet inhibition • Neutropenia	• NSAIDs should be avoided in patients with platelet dysfunction or thrombocytopenia (<50,000) • Neutropenia incidence <1%
Renal	• AKI • Chronic renal failure	• AKI from hemodynamic injury typically occurs within the first week of NSAID therapy; occurs in patients dependent on prostaglandin for renal perfusion (i.e., renal insufficiency or effective volume depletion); low-dose aspirin and ibuprofen have lower risk; NSAIDs more rarely cause AKI secondary to interstitial nephritis • Chronic kidney disease associated with high-dose and long-duration NSAID therapy
Skin	• Rash • Stevens–Johnson syndrome, toxic epidermal necrolysis	

TABLE 14.1.3 Adjuvant Analgesics

Drug	Syndrome	Dosing	Comments
Anticonvulsants			
Gabapentin: 100, 300, 400 mg caps; 600, 800 mg tabs; 250 mg/5mL PO solution	Neuropathic pain	Initial 100 mg PO TID increase by 100 mg TID Q 3 days; 300–3,600 mg/day divided TID	Adjust dose for renal dysfunction (CrCl <60 mL/min); no significant documented drug-drug interactions; do not stop abruptly; monitor for changes in mood, suicidal ideation
Pregabalin (Lyrica): 25, 50, 75, 100, 150, 200, 225, 300 mg caps	Neuropathic pain	Initial 150 mg PO divided BID/TID; max 450 mg divided BID/TID	
Lamotrigine (Lamictal): 25, 50, 100, 200 mg tabs; 2, 5, 25 mg chewable tabs; 25, 50, 100, 200, 300 mg XR tabs; 25, 50, 100 mg ODTs	Neuropathic pain	Initial 25 mg QOD 2 weeks; then 25 mg QD 2 weeks; then by 25–50 mg/day Q 1–2 weeks; up to 50–400 mg/day typical	Do not discontinue abruptly
Topiramate (Topamax): 15, 25 mg sprinkle caps; 25, 50, 100, 200 mg tabs	Neuropathic pain	Initial 25–50 mg QD; ↑ by 25–50 mg Q week; 200 mg BID studied; max 1,600 mg/day	Limited data
Valproic acid: 125, 250, 500 mg softgel IR and XR; 250/5 mL PO solution	Neuropathic pain	Initial 125 mg TID; maint; 500–1,000 mg TID	Monitor levels (<100 µg/mL); CYP-450 inhibitor; monitor for drug interactions
Antidepressants			
Duloxetine (Cymbalta): 20, 30, 60 mg caps	Diabetic neuropathy, fibromyalgia	Initial 20 mg daily initial; typical 20–60 mg/day (QD or divide BID)	May increase BP; monitor for changes in mood, suicidal ideation
Venlafaxine (Effexor): 25, 37.5, 50, 75, 100 mg tabs; 37.5, 50, 75, 150, 225 mg XR tabs; 37.5, 50, 75, 150 mg XR caps	Neuropathic pain	Initial 37.5–75 mg/day; may ↑ dose Q 4 days by 75 mg/day; typical 75–225 mg/day divided BID/TID	Causes increased BP; monitor
Amitriptyline: 10, 25, 50, 75, 100, 150 mg tabs Nortriptyline: 10, 25, 50, 75 mg caps; 10 mg/5 mL PO solution Desipramine: 10, 25, 50, 75, 100, 150 mg tabs	Neuropathic pain	Initial 25 mg PO HS; 10 mg if frail, elderly; typical 25–100 mg HS; 1–2 weeks (up to 4) for effects; titrate every few days to ↓ adverse effects	Anticholinergic effects increased with SSRIs; avoid tramadol: due to ↑ seizure risk; anticholinergic effects: amitriptyline >nortriptyline >desipramine

(Continued)

TABLE 14.1.3 Adjuvant Analgesics *(Continued)*

Drug	Syndrome	Dosing	Comments
Corticosteroids			
Dexamethasone: 0.5, 0.75, 1, 1.5, 2, 4, 6 mg tabs; 0.5/5 mL, 1 mg/30 mL PO solution; solution for injection	Spinal cord compression, ↑ ICP	Load 40–100 mg IV dex or equivalent (methylprednisolone 40–80 mg IV) or 10–20 mg IV Q 6 for initial 24–72h	High dose ≤72 h; if no benefit, dose can be rapidly tapered; if pain improves, taper to lowest effective dose
Methylprednisolone: 4, 8, 16, 32 mg tabs; solution and suspension for injection	Nerve compression, visceral distension, ↑ ICP	Dex 4–8 mg PO Q 8–12 h; methylprednisolone 20–40 mg PO Q 8–12 h	Usefulness limited to 2–3 months before steroid-induced side effects outweigh benefit
	Bone pain, nausea, anorexia	Dex 4–12 mg/day	
Other			
Lidocaine patch (Lidoderm) 5%	Postherpetic neuralgia	1 patch for 12hr/day; 1–3 patches	Clinical experience supports use in painful peripheral neuralgia
Pamidronate (Aredia): 3, 6, 9 mg/mL injection solution; 30, 90 mg powder for reconstitution	Bone pain	90 mg IV Q 4 weeks, may ↓ interval to Q 3 weeks; ↓ dose renal dysfunction	Decreased impact of disease progression in patients with osteolytic lesions secondary to multiple myeloma, breast cancer, prostate cancer
Zoledronic acid (Zometa, Reclast): 4, 5 mg/ 100 mL, 4 mg/5 mL injection solution		4 mg IV Q 4 weeks; may ↓ interval to Q 3 weeks; ↓ dose renal dysfunction	

Reproduced with permission from Scullion BF, Ryan L. Pain. In: Attridge R, Miller M, Moote R, Ryan L, eds. *Internal Medicine: A Guide to Clinical Therapeutics*. New York, NY: McGraw-Hill; 2012:chap 45. Table 45-3.

TABLE 14.2.1 Suggested Opioid Regimens by Clinical Situation

Situation	Opioid Regimen
Acute episodic pain in opioid naïve patient	• Provide short-acting IV or PO opioid on PRN basis (see Table 14.2.2) • Monitor pain response and increase dose or consider scheduling opioid if pain poorly controlled
Acute severe pain in opioid naïve patient	• Morphine 1–5 mg IV (or equivalent dose of another opioid) • Reassess pain in 15 min; if pain level has not dropped 2–4 points on VAS, then double morphine dose • Repeat for 1 more cycle if pain uncontrolled • Monitor respiratory rate and sensorium closely; have naloxone available • Schedule an appropriate opioid regimen once acute control achieved
Chronic pain in opioid naïve patient	• Schedule either short-acting or long-acting opioid at appropriate dosing intervals (see Table 14.2.2) • Provide PRN opioid for breakthrough pain; rule of thumb is to provide breakthrough dose equivalent to 10–15% of the total daily scheduled regimen (per dose) • Example: Morphine CR 15 mg Q 12 h and morphine IR 5 mg Q 4 h PRN
Uncontrolled pain in a patient already taking opioids	• Mild-to-moderate pain: increase total daily opioid dose by 25–50% • Moderate-to-severe pain: increase total daily opioid dose by 50–100% • May increase dose every 24 h
Decreased opioid dose required in patient on chronic opioids	• Dose de-escalation may be required due to adverse effects; introduction of an adjunctive pain medicine or patient undergoing pain relief procedure • Reduce scheduled opioid dose by 30–50% and monitor patient

Sources: (1) McPherson, MLM. *Demystifying Opioid Conversion Calculations: A Guide for Effective Dosing.* Bethesda, MD: American Society of Health-System Pharmacists; 2009. (2) Weissman DE. *Opioid Dose Escalation,* 2nd ed. Fast Facts and Concepts. July 2005; 20. http://www.eperc.mcw.edu/fastfact/ff_020.htm

TABLE 14.2.2 Opioid Dosing in Naïve Patients

Drug	Products	Typical Dosing	Onset	Duration	Comments
Oral Short-Acting Opioids					
Codeine	15, 30, 60 mg	30 mg PO Q 4–6 h	30 min	4–6 h	• Total daily dose limited by acetaminophen content; do not exceed 4 g acetaminophen per day; avoid in liver disease
Hydrocodone	Only available combined with acetaminophen or ibuprofen at various doses	5–10 mg PO Q 4 h	30 min	4 h	
Hydromorphone	2, 4, 8 mg	2–4 mg PO Q 4 h	30 min	4 h	
Morphine	10, 15, 30 mg	15 mg PO Q 4 h	30 min	4 h	
Oxycodone	5, 10, 15, 20, 30 mg	5–10 mg PO Q 4 h	30 min	4 h	• Also available in various combinations with acetaminophen
Oxymorphone	5, 10 mg	5–10 mg PO Q 4–6 h	1 h	4–6 h	
Tapentadol (Nucynta)	50, 75, 100 mg	50 mg PO Q 4–6 h	30–60 min	4–6 h	
Tramadol	50 mg	50 mg PO Q 6 h	30–60 min	4–6 h	
Parenteral Opioids					
Buprenorphine	0.3 mg/mL	0.3 mg IV Q 6 h		6 h	• Partial mu agonist, can cause withdrawal if given to opioid-dependent patients
Fentanyl	0.05 mg/mL	0.05–0.1 mg IV/SC Q 1–2 h	Immediate	1–2 h	
Hydromorphone	1 mg/mL	0.5–1 IV mg Q 4 h	5–10 min	2–4 h	
Methadone	10 mg/mL	2.5 mg IV/SC Q 4–8 h	10–20 min	4–6 h	• IV methadone is twice as potent as oral
Morphine	Various strengths: 0.5–50 mg/mL	2–5 mg IV/SC Q 2–4 h	5–10 min	2–4 h	
Oxymorphone	1 mg/mL	0.5 IV/SC Q 4–6 h	5–10 min	3–6 h	

Oral Long-Acting Opioids					
Hydromorphone ER (Exalgo)	8, 12, 18 mg	8 mg PO QD		24 h	
Morphine CR	15, 30, 60, 100, 200 mg	15 mg PO Q 12 h		8–12 h	
Morphine ER (Kadian, Avinza)	Kadian: 10, 20, 30, 50, 60, 80, 100, 200 mg Avinza: 30, 45, 60, 75, 90, 120 mg	10–30 mg PO QD		24 h	• Kadian may last <24 h, may give Q 12 h • May sprinkle capsule contents on applesauce or give via G-tube; instruct patient not to chew beads in applesauce • Do not coadminister Avinza with alcohol
Oxycodone CR (OxyContin)	10, 15, 20, 30, 40, 60 80 mg	10 mg PO Q 12 h		8–12 h	
Methadone	5, 10, 40 mg tablets 5, 10 mg/mL solution	2.5–5 mg Q 4–8 h 2.5 mg Q 12–24 in elderly patients	10–15 min	4–8 h	• Methadone has a long half-life but a clinically short duration until sufficient accumulation in 4–7 days • One titration method is to initiate 5–10 mg Q 4 PRN for 7 days, then convert to BID or TID scheduled regimen equal to total methadone requirement on day 7
Tapentadol ER (Nucynta ER)	50, 100, 150, 200, 250 mg	50 mg PO QD		24 h	
Tramadol ER (Ultram ER)	100, 200, 300 mg	100 mg PO QD		24 h	

TABLE 14.2.3 Opioid Equianalgesic Dose Conversions

Drug	Equianalgesic Dose (mg)		Stepwise Conversion Procedure
	Oral	Parenteral	
Morphine	30	10	• Calculate total 24-h opioid dose of each different opioid being taken
Hydromorphone	7.5	1.5	• Convert total 24-h dose of each opioid to an equivalent dose in oral morphine equivalents using the table.
Oxycodone	20	—	Add equivalent doses of each opioid being taken together to get the total daily oral morphine equivalent dose
Hydrocodone	30	—	• Determine the dose of the new opioid regimen equal to the calculated daily oral morphine equivalent using
Oxymorphone	10	1	the table
Fentanyl	—	0.1 (100 µg)	• Reduce calculated dose of new opioid by 25–50% to prevent overdose from incomplete cross-tolerance
Meperidine	300	75	between opioids
Tramadol	120	—	
Buprenorphine	0.4	0.3	

TABLE 14.2.4 Fentanyl Transdermal Patch Conversions

Fentanyl TDS (g/h)	Morphine (mg/day)		Stepwise Conversion Procedures
	PO	IV	
25	50	17	*Conversion from another opioid regimen to fentanyl TDS*
50	100	33	1. Calculate total daily dose of opioid including long- and short-acting agents
75	150	50	2. Use conversion chart (Table 14.2.1) to convert; total daily dose to oral morphine equivalents
100	200	67	3. Convert oral morphine equivalents to fentanyl TDS and round to patch size per individual patient
125	250	83	characteristics:
150	300	100	• Round down if patient is elderly, has renal or liver impairment, or was well controlled on prior regimen
175	350	117	• Round up if pain control was inadequate on previous regimen
200	400	133	4. Perceptible analgesia is delayed 12 h and peak analgesia occurs around 36 h after patch application
225	450	150	• Give prior long-acting opioid for the first 12 h and short-acting breakthrough doses until pain controlled.
250	500	167	*Conversion from fentanyl TDS to another opioid regimen*
275	550	183	• Use conversion chart to determine daily oral morphine equivalent dose to fentanyl TDS
300	600	200	• Construct logical equivalent oral or IV opioid regimen as per clinical situation
			• Fentanyl will be absorbed from the skin in gradually decreasing quantities for 24 h after patch removal.
			Delay initiation of new scheduled regimen for 12–24 h and provide short-acting opioids for breakthrough

Sources: (1) ScullionBF, Ryan L. Pain. In: Attridge R, Miller M, Moote R, Ryan L, eds. *Internal Medicine: A Guide to Clinical Therapeutics.* New York, NY: McGraw-Hill;2012:chap 45. (2) McPherson, MLM. Transdermal and parenteral fentanyl dosage calculations and conversions. In: *Demystifying Opioid Conversion Calculations: A Guide for Effective Dosing.* Bethesda, MD: American Society of Health-System Pharmacists;2009:chap 5. (3) Weissman DE. *Converting to/from Transdermal Fentanyl.* 2nd ed. Fast Facts and Concepts. July 2005; 2. http://www.eperc.mcw.edu/fastfact/ff_002.htm

TABLE 14.2.5　Methadone Conversions

Total Daily Oral Morphine Equivalent Dose (mg)	Oral Morphine:Methadone Equivalent Daily Dose (mg:mg)	Comments
<100	4:1	• Conversion from morphine to methadone is complex and highly variable from patient to patient
101–300	8:1	• The conversion is not linear; higher daily doses of morphine (or equivalent) require lower doses of methadone on a mg per mg basis
301–600	10:1	• This table reflects one of several published conversion ratios; these ratios are more conservative than many others in the literature
601–800	12:1	
801–1,000	15:1	
>1,000	20:1	

Stepwise Conversion Procedure (Using Ratios)

1. Add total 24-h opioid dose of each different opioid being taken
2. Convert total 24-h dose of each opioid to an equivalent dose in oral morphine equivalents using the table. Add equivalent doses of each opioid being taken together to get the total daily oral morphine equivalent dose
3. Convert total daily oral morphine equivalent dose to methadone dose using above ratios
4. Reduce calculated dose of methadone by 30–50% to account for incomplete cross-tolerance. Give in divided dose Q 8 h

Alternative Conversion Procedure

1. Follow steps 1 and 2 of the stepwise conversion procedure
2. Convert total daily morphine equivalent dose to methadone dose using 10:1 ratio (or 20:1 ratio if patient >65 years old or daily morphine >1,000 mg)
3. Give calculated methadone dose (up to 30 mg) every 3 h PRN
4. Continue for 6 days. After 6 days, average total methadone requirement from day 5 and 6. This average dose is the new daily scheduled dose of methadone (divided BID)

Sources: (1) Scullion BF, Ryan L. Pain. In: Attridge R, Miller M, Moote R, Ryan L, eds. *Internal Medicine: A Guide to Clinical Therapeutics.* New York, NY: McGraw-Hill;2012:chap 45. (2) McPherson, MLM. Methadone: A Complex and Challenging Analgesic, But Its Worth It. In: *Demystifying Opioid Conversion Calculations: A Guide for Effective Dosing.* Bethesda, MD: American Society of Health-System Pharmacists;2009:chap 6. (3) Gazelle G, Fine PG. *Methadone for the Treatment of Pain.* 2nd ed. Fast Facts and Concepts. July 2006; 75. http://www.eperc.mcw.edu/fastfact/ff_075.htm

TABLE 14.2.6 Opioid Adverse Effects

Effected System	Symptoms	Comments
Cardiovascular	• Hypotension (more common with IV push opioids) • QTc prolongation (methadone)	• Cardiac monitoring for methadone: obtain ECG at baseline, at 30 days and annually, at 30 days and annually, inform patient of risks, discontinue if QTc >500 ms, check for interacting drugs (*Ann Int Med.* 2009;150:387)
Central nervous system (CNS)	• Withdrawal: mydriasis, diaphoresis, tachycardia, anxiety, hypertension • CNS depression: sedation, somnolence, confusion • Other: euphoria, confusion, delirium, hallucinations	• Patients receiving continuous opioids for 1–2 weeks are at risk of withdrawal if opioid discontinued • Onset usually 6–12 h after last dose (short-acting opioid) or 72–96 h following methadone • Can avoid withdrawal by tapering by 25% every 2 days
Gastrointestinal	Nausea, vomiting, constipation	• Patients taking scheduled opioids should be on a scheduled bowel regimen including a stimulant laxative (typically Senna) to prevent constipation
Respiratory	Respiratory depression: may have frequent shallow breaths initially, followed by decreased respiratory rate or apnea	• Respiratory depression is preceded by CNS depression, sedation, somnolence or miosis; should be considered a warning sign for impending respiratory depression
Skin	Pruritus	• Related to histamine release; morphine, codeine and meperidine tend to be more histaminic than other opioids
Urinary tract	Urinary retention, difficulty voiding	

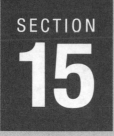

SECTION 15

Urology

ABBREVIATIONS			
BPH	Benign prostatic hyperplasia	PSA	Prostate-specific antigen
IR	Immediate release	XR	Extended release

FIGURE 15.1.1 Treatment Algorithm for BPH

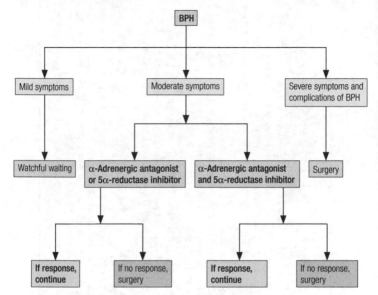

Reproduced with permission from Talbert RL, DiPiro JT, Matzke GR, Posey LM, Wells BG, Yee GC.
Benign Prostatic Hyperplasia. In: Talbert RL, DiPiro JT, Matzke GR, Posey LM, Wells BG, Yee GC, eds.
Pharmacotherapy: A Pathophysiologic Approach. 8th ed. New York, NY: McGraw-Hill; 2011:chap 93

TABLE 15.1.2 Pharmacotherapy for BPH

Drug	Dosing	Peak Onset	Comments
Nonselective α-Adrenergic Antagonists			
Alfuzosin (Uroxatral)	10 mg QD	1 week	• Orthostatic hypotension, syncope and dizziness common with doxazosin, prazosin and terazosin; in particular with the first few doses; 10% of patients will stop taking due to side effects (*Int J Clin Pract.* 2008;62:1547); start with low dose and titrate up as tolerated over the course of 4–6 weeks
Doxazosin (Cardura)	1–8 mg QD	2–6 weeks	• Prazosin not recommended due to more side effects (*J Urol.* 2003;170:530)
Doxazosin GTS (Cardura XL)	4–8 mg QD	1 week	• Alfuzosin has a low incidence of cardiovascular side effects due to its low serum and high prostate concentration: dose titration is not needed
Prazosin (Minipress)	0.5–2 mg BID	2–6 weeks	• These agents will not effect PSA, prostate size, or alter disease progression
Terazosin (Hytrin)	1–10 mg QD	2–6 weeks	
Selective α-Adrenergic Antagonists			
Silodosin (Rapaflo)	8 mg QD	1 week	• Tamsulosin and silodosin have low incidence of cardiovascular side effects
Tamsulosin (Flomax)	0.4–0.8 mg QD	1 week	• Common side effects include flu-like illness, fatigue, nasal congestion, and ejaculatory dysfunction
5α-Reductase Inhibitors			
Dutasteride (Avodart)	0.5 mg QD	3–6 months	• Sexual side effects occur in approximately 10% of patients and include erectile dysfunction, ejaculatory dysfunction, and decreased libido
Finasteride (Proscar)	5 mg QD	3–6 months	• Will reduce prostate size and PSA; measured PSA should be doubled to reflect true value in patients taking these agents (*J Urol.* 2003;170:530)
			• Finasteride and dutasteride reduced prostate cancer incidence by ~25% over 7 and 4 years, respectively (*N Engl J Med.* 2003;349:215; *N Engl J Med.* 2010;362:1192)

TABLE 15.2.1 Pharmacotherapy of Urinary Incontinence

Drug	Indications	Dosing	Comments
Antimuscarinic Agents			
Darifenacin (Enablex)	Urge incontinence	7.5–15 mg QD	• Antimuscarinics are first-line therapy for urge incontinence
Fesoterodine (Toviaz)	Urge incontinence	4–8 mg QD	• A systematic review of comparative trials found that tolterodine IR was better tolerated than oxybutynin IR; solifenacin and fesoterodine had better efficacy than tolterodine XR, but fesoterodine had higher incidence of adverse effects (*Cochrane Database Syst Rev.* 2012;1:CD005429)
Oxybutynin (Ditropan, Anturol, Gelnique, Oxytrol)	Urge incontinence	IR (Ditropan): 2.5–5 mg BID-QID XR (Ditropan XL): 5–30 mg QD Patch (Oxytrol): 3.9 mg patch applied Q 3–4 days Gel (Gelnique): One sachet applied QD Gel (Anturol): 84 mg (3 pumps) applied QD	• Dry mouth, constipation, dizziness, and visual disturbances are common, highest incidence with oxybutynin IR and tolterodine IR, lowest incidence with oxybutynin patch and gel and solifenacin
Tolterodine (Detrol)	Urge incontinence	IR (Detrol): 1–2 mg BID XR (Detrol LA): 2–4 mg QD	• Patients with dementia taking a cholinesterase inhibitor will have greater decline in function if also taking an antimuscarinic (*Drugs Aging.* 2003;20:437)
Trospium (Sanctura, generics)	Urge incontinence	60 mg QD	
Solifenacin (Vesicare)	Urge incontinence	5–10 mg QD	

(Continued)

TABLE 15.2.1 Pharmacotherapy of Urinary Incontinence (Continued)

Drug	Indications	Dosing	Comments
Antidepressants			
Duloxetine (Cymbalta)	Stress incontinence	40–80 mg QD	• Anticholinergic side effects (dry mouth, dizziness, constipation) and orthostasis common with imipramine; start at low dose and take at night to minimize
Imipramine	Urge incontinence, stress incontinence	25–100 mg QHS	• Nausea common with duloxetine; improves over time • Both agents have modest efficacy
α-Adrenergic Agonists			
Pseudoephedrine	Stress incontinence	15–60 mg TID	• Avoid in patients with hypertension, ischemic heart disease, arrhythmias, or renal failure
Phenylephrine	Stress incontinence	10 mg QID	
Cholinomimetic			
Bethanechol	Atonic bladder	25–50 mg TID–QID	• Take on empty stomach

INDEX